TRIUMPH

Getting Back to Normal When You Have Cancer

Other Avon Books by
Marion Morra and Eve Potts

CHOICES: REALISTIC ALTERNATIVES IN CANCER TREATMENT
(An Avon Books Trade Paperback)

UNDERSTANDING YOUR IMMUNE SYSTEM

TRIUMPH

Getting Back to Normal When You Have Cancer

MARION MORRA and **EVE POTTS**

AVON BOOKS ◆ NEW YORK

This book was current to the best of the authors' knowledge at publication, but before acting on information herein the consumer should, of course, verify information with the appropriate physician or agency.

TRIUMPH: GETTING BACK TO NORMAL WHEN YOU HAVE CANCER is an original publication of Avon Books. This work has never before appeared in book form.

AVON BOOKS
A division of
The Hearst Corporation
105 Madison Avenue
New York, New York 10016

First Avon Books Trade Printing: February 1990

AVON TRADEMARK REG. U.S. PAT. OFF. AND IN OTHER COUNTRIES, MARCA REGISTRADA, HECHO EN U.S.A.

Printed in the U.S.A.

OPM 10 9 8 7 6 5 4 3 2 1

To the many people with cancer
who inspired us,
and to our wonderful supportive family
who made it possible
for us to write this book.

Acknowledgments

This book is dedicated to all the patients, physicians, and researchers who are responsible for the remarkable new "triumphant" attitudes toward cancer. We thank the hundreds of people across the country who shared their experiences with us both in person and by letter. It is their life experiences, along with the latest research findings presented in medical and psychological journals and at medical conferences, that have served as sources of information for this book.

We are indebted to the excellent staff at the Cancer Information Office of the Yale Comprehensive Cancer Center for its unstinting dedication and help, and to the M.D. Anderson Cancer Center's public relations staff who distributed our questionnaires to patients and their families.

We are especially grateful to Judith Riven, Executive Editor, Avon Books, who lent new insights and clarity to this endeavor. Last but not least, very special thanks to Robert Potts for his never-ending patience, understanding, and good humor, and to the rest of our families for their continuing help and support.

Contents

Preface

Ever since we began researching our first book on cancer, *CHOICES: Realistic Alternatives in Cancer Treatment* (Avon Books, 1980 and 1987), we have been struck by the ever-increasing number of people we know who have triumphed over cancer. We've watched them swing back into action, taking treatment in stride, putting the cancer experience into perspective, and going on with their lives. We noticed that along the way to becoming triumphers, certain patterns were evident. After an initial period when minds go into low gear, decisions are difficult to make, and dependency on doctors and other caretakers becomes the order of the day, focus begins to change. Gradually, one learns to live with the idea of having cancer, becomes aggressive about looking at the mountains of material available on cancer, and learns to make sense of it, picking up clues to serve as guidelines, acting on treatments, thinking through options. Once past the "sickness state," we've watched new determination shift into high gear and a whole new, learned perception of image and future emerge from the search—and a wiser, healthier life begin to evolve.

It is clear that today's cancer triumphers differ from cancer patients of other times. Most *expect* to survive—understanding that cancer is a chronic disease. Instead of resigning themselves to what used to be considered a fatal illness, many, after the initial period of shock, set out readjusting, exploring, and fighting for their lives. They schedule their treatments so that they do not interfere with their daily schedules. They plan chemo treatments for week's end so they can go home afterward without disrupting their work schedules. Life goes on with new zest. They travel. They savor each moment. They live full, active lives.

Triumphers know the importance of "shopping" for doctors and treatment centers—demanding compassionate attitudes as well as the very best of medical expertise. Even what used to be considered suspect and nontraditional therapies have come under new scrutiny and some, like mind-control therapies and diet, nutrition and vitamin therapy, have been included as a part of the normal arsenal of treatment. As we all come to understand ourselves and our bodies better, as the medical profession continues to broaden the variety of options available and past stigmas are erased, anxieties and tensions, problems and hurdles are accepted and understood, and self-reliance and a feeling of well-being and triumph prevail.

We hope the facts and information in *TRIUMPH: Getting Back to Normal When You Have Cancer* will help to provide a broad map back to good health. Naturally, since this book is designed as a health-education service, it is not intended as a substitute for medical advice from physicians or health professionals.

Put These Thoughts into Your Mental Computer

- People have recovered from every type of cancer.
- Cancer is the most curable of all chronic diseases.
- Cancer patients can expect to live longer than either heart attack or stroke victims.
- A positive attitude helps let go of stress and worry.
- It helps to learn about every detail of your kind of cancer.
- A fighting spirit is healthier than stoic acceptance.
- Many patients whom doctors consider difficult are those who are most likely to get well.
- A fighting spirit can strengthen your immune response.
- It's better to express your feelings than to bottle them up.
- Hope and trust help counteract stress.
- Stress comes from your own interpretation of events.
- Hope gives you control.
- Refusal to hope is a decision to die.
- Consider yourself an equal partner with your doctor in achieving recovery.
- Listen to your body.
- Remember you have power over your body.
- Don't make a career of having cancer.
- Don't save up real living for tomorrow. Live your best today.

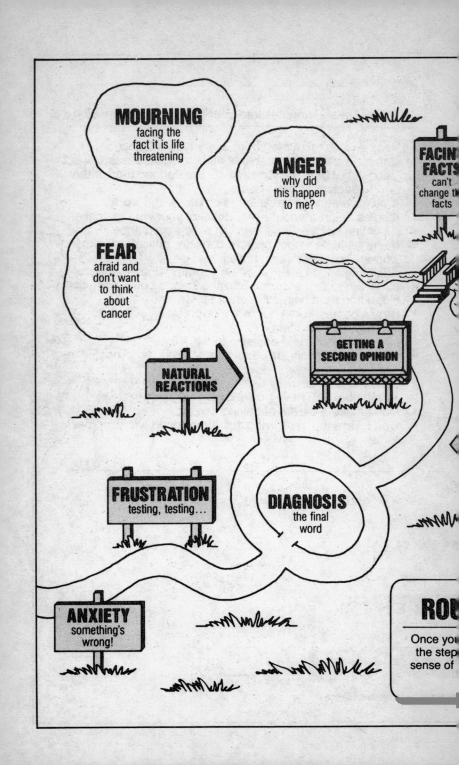

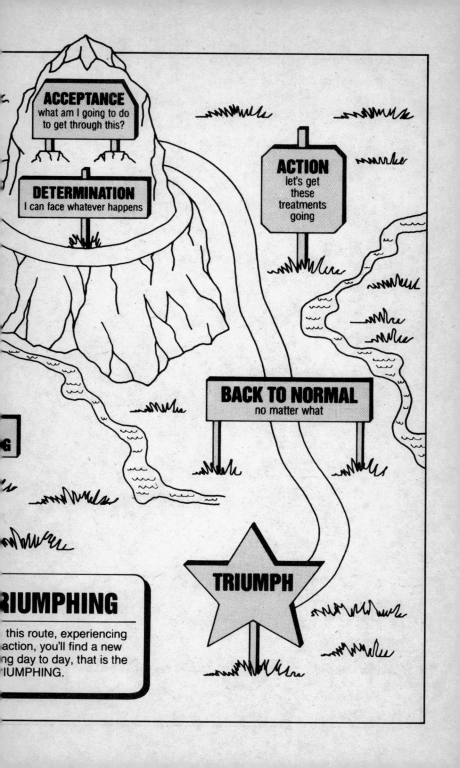

ACCEPTANCE
what am I going to do to get through this?

DETERMINATION
I can face whatever happens

ACTION
let's get these treatments going

BACK TO NORMAL
no matter what

TRIUMPH

RIUMPHING

this route, experiencing action, you'll find a new g day to day, that is the IUMPHING.

TRIUMPH

Getting Back to Normal When You Have Cancer

chapter 1

Facing What's Happened

First, let's try to strip away all the old myths about cancer —myths that have come down to us through family stories and old wives' tales. Whispered conversations that somehow indicated there was something sinister or even vaguely "dirty" about having cancer used to set the stage for hiding the diagnosis from the patient as well as from friends. The "fear" word CANCER never was uttered. Things have changed a lot—but many of the old fears remain.

Let's take a look at some of the stumbling blocks that still stand in the way of psychological recovery of cancer patients. Many of those who know the cancer patient, no matter what they've been told of the diagnosis, often take a wait-and-see attitude. They may avoid seeing you and talking about your problems. They may seem oversolicitous about your health. They may treat you as though you're wrapped in cotton batting. Their concern is rooted in worry for your health, but it can come through to you as an uncomfortable feeling that they don't quite believe you're really going to get better. Exploring their feelings and your own is important and can be very helpful in clearing the air. The feedback you may get from friends, family, and employers which may give you the nagging feeling they aren't sure about your recovery also explains why cancer patients so often feel the need to act as cheerleaders, always keeping up a good front so that everyone really will believe they're going to get better. It puts a terrible strain on you, the person who is trying to recover.

How do you deal with all this? Decide at the outset that you will not make a career out of having cancer. After all, before you discovered you had cancer, you played other roles in life. You're a mother, a father, a daughter, a son, a wife, a husband. You are involved in a career, a profession, school, homemaking, or other activity. You are an important part of a group of friends. You golf, play tennis, root for your favorite team. Don't let cancer and cancer treatments take over your life. Get some part of your life back to true normal immediately. Don't let anything or anyone force you into making your entire life the patient role. Your illness is just one part of your existence. Get on with thinking about other things. Try to keep a perspective on your life so you can go forward with the business of living.

What does cured mean?

Cured means that you have the same life expectancy as someone your age who never had cancer. *Cancer is, in fact, the most curable of all chronic diseases. Latest statistics show that about 60 percent of all serious cancers can be cured.*

"The first time I went to the hospital for treatment I met a woman who had been treated for the same thing I had and was there for a 10-year checkup. I realized then that cancer is not an automatic death sentence. Do your homework, get as much information as you can and more than one opinion."

Diagnosed with non-Hodgkin's lymphoma in 1986 at age 54

What is meant by the chronic nature of cancer?

Some of the chronic aspects of cancer have to do with the nature of the disease. Others have to do with the treatments that are used to rid the body of cancer. A chronic disease differs from a fatal disease in that it has continuing problems, all of which can be handled. Diabetes, for example, is a chronic disease that once was considered a fatal disease. A fatal disease is one in which the disease process cannot be slowed and which, in a short period of time, kills. Cancer used to be considered a fatal disease. Today, it is viewed as a chronic disease. So, adjust your thinking to encompass that fact.

How do cancer statistics compare with the statistics for stroke and heart disease?

An amazing fact becomes apparent when you look at the statistics. Cancer patients can expect to live longer than either stroke or heart attack victims. At least half of stroke patients die within the first year and 30 percent of heart attack patients do not survive their initial convalescent period. Many cancer patients, on the other hand, are cured and can expect to live normal life spans. More than half of all cancer patients can expect to live for at least five years—usually much more. That's why it is very important for you to aim at achieving a lifestyle that returns you to normal living as quickly as possible.

What about statistics that show that my odds of beating cancer aren't all that good?

Statistics are based on large groups of patients of different ages—some of whom have been diagnosed early, some who were diagnosed late in the course of their disease. Some receive the ultimate in care, others receive a minimal amount of adequate care. There are many other variables. Some have a strong will to live, others are ready to die. No matter what the statistics say, there are people with your kind of cancer who have succeeded in being cured. Decide that you'll be in that category of the statistics.

Don't Let Survival Statistics Undo You

Don't be misled by statistics on survival times and rates of recurrence. Your physician may talk to you about "five-year survival" rates. Many people misinterpret this to mean that you are expected to live only five years after treatment or that you aren't considered cured. Five-year survival is used as a measure by scientists for patients who have cancer to compare the value of one treatment against another. Statistics are gathered for a five-year period. In many forms of cancer, five years without symptoms following treatment is the accepted time to consider a patient cured. However, depending on the type of cancer, some patients are considered cured after one year, others after three years, while for some it may be five years and longer.

Why do people treat their fear of cancer differently from their fears of other life-threatening diseases?

Most people do not realize how deeply their fears are rooted in outdated facts about cancer. The reasons for fear are many. They are varied and complex. They are the result of traumatic experiences that have been observed with others who have had cancer. They are rooted in our literature and media that continually refer to uncontrollable situations as "cancerous." Fear of cancer—the fear that you are losing control over your body and your life—is much like the fear of flying, the fear of not being certain whether you'll finish the flight alive.

How can I cope with my very real fears about not recovering from cancer?

The first step is to search your fears. The minute you start worrying about cancer, practice acknowledging your fears and remind yourself that you can alter your own reactions to those fears. Consider reprogramming your thinking with new information about the success of many cancer treatments. Your own thoughts, programmed to positive facts about how cancer is being cured today, will start to create positive feelings to replace the negative ones. Simplistic as this sounds, it is an effective way to start changing your reaction to your illness. It's important that you try not to suppress your negative feelings. That will only succeed in pushing them further into your unconscious where they will reappear to haunt you with even more vengeance in the future. Ignoring or suppressing your fears will only magnify them.

"Medical attention is the crucial basis for recovery—but the patient must play his role as well. Cancer is an obstacle in life which some of us have been chosen to face, unfortunately. Cancer threatens our lives. I was scared and frightened that I would die. I was mad and could not understand why it happened to me. But this initial feeling must be overcome in order to win. It is so very hard to conquer the fear of death, but with understanding, education, support, faith, time, and the willingness to FIGHT, you can win."

Diagnosed with osteosarcoma in 1984 at age 16

How much should I be telling other people about what's happening to me?

The advice of most triumphers is to share the diagnosis with family and friends—and to do it from the very beginning. Don't be afraid to discuss what you've been told. Don't try to hide from the diagnosis. This is the time when you need the support of everyone around you to help you in your fight to get through to full recovery. You will probably find that the more open you are with others, the less frightened you will be. Your strength will be conveyed to others who usually will be able to be more supportive of you. This exchange can help to build a very positive atmosphere.

Explore Your Feelings

Ask yourself:
What am I most afraid of?
   Pain?
   Losing control of my life?
   Not being able to cope?
   Facing the fact that I may die?

What triggers my fears and makes them worse?
   Reading cancer statistics?
   Talking about my cancer experience?
   Going for treatments?
   Going for checkups?
   Middle-of-the-night worries?

What makes me feel more in control?
   Knowing everything there is to know about my kind of cancer and treatment?
   Talking about my fears?
   Dealing with my fears through relaxation techniques?
   Doing something that takes my mind off the whole subject?

How much do I really want to know about what's wrong with me?

The answer depends on how you cope with problems. Most people cope best with full information. Often, this information is shared with someone close who can help in the information-gathering task. It is helpful to learn as much as you can about the kind of cancer you have and about the treatments that are available to help cure it. Arming yourself with knowledge will go a long way in alleviating your worries, doubts, and fears. It's the NOT KNOWING that raises questions and builds worrying barriers.

What if I feel uncertain about whether I have the right doctor and the right hospital?

Part of the educational process of dealing with cancer, and an important part of the process of recovering, has to do with learning absolutely everything you can about your kind of cancer. There are a number of steps involved—and you don't have to feel that you must take these all by yourself. You can enlist family and friends to help.

First of all, you must read as much as you can of the medical literature by the foremost people in the field—getting and grasping the facts about your cancer. The best place to start to gather this information is by making a call to the 1-800-4-CANCER number, the Cancer Information Service. This service, backed by the formidable knowledge of the National Cancer Institute, the federal government's principal agency for research on cancer, is staffed with knowledgeable people who will take the time to assist you personally in getting the information you need to make decisions. The range of information you can ask from them includes:

- Any pamphlets or booklets of the National Cancer Institute which discusses your kind of cancer.
- PDQ computer information sheets. (PDQ, which stands for Physician Data Query, is a computerized system that

gives the latest state-of-the-art information compiled by
leading physicians across the country on treatments recommended for each kind of cancer.)

- Information on medical journal articles on your cancer.
- Information on leading physicians and hospitals where
  your kind of cancer is being treated.

---

*"The most important thing is to seek the best
treatment you can get, preferably at a Cancer
Center. Do not passively rely on your friendly
family doctor. Many doctors are not up on
technology and treatments. You deserve the
best."*

Diagnosed with breast cancer in 1978 at age 57

What is the proper way to ask for a second or third opinion?

Many people are squeamish about telling their doctors that
they want other opinions before going ahead with treatments
or with making changes at any time during treatment. You
need not be. Getting other opinions about a medical problem is a prudent procedure—and important before making
irreversible decisions. You can proceed in one of two ways.
You can ask your doctor to help you in finding other physicians who can assess your case or, even better, you can take
things into your own hands and make appointments for yourself with physicians who are experts in the area of your kind
of cancer. If you do your homework, you can make your own
judgments about which doctors you would like to have consider your case. Don't hesitate to make personal phone calls
to physicians whose medical writings you feel have a bearing
on your case. Most are willing to take calls and give information over the phone.

Another choice is to make an appointment with the specialists at the nearest Comprehensive Cancer Center. There
are 20 Comprehensive Cancer Centers in the United States,

designated by the National Cancer Institute. They vary from centers that treat only cancer patients to centers in medical schools or in community hospitals. All are well known for their expertise either in cancer research, patient care, or both. They are specifically geared to treating cancer with the most up-to-date methods. Listings of all Comprehensive Cancer Centers are included in Chapter 9.

Thought:

NOT MAKING A DECISION IS ANOTHER WAY OF MAKING A DECISION

Why is it important for me that my doctor be an oncologist?

An oncologist is a doctor who is an expert in dealing with cancer patients. You should look for an internist who is a specialist in medical oncology as your doctor. There are also surgical oncologists, radiation oncologists, and gynecological oncologists. These are physicians who have made treating cancer their life's work, and are up to date about the latest methods of treating the disease. Don't make the assumption that every doctor who deals with cancer patients is so equipped. Check out your doctor's credentials with care.

Is it usual to see a change in relationships with people when you have cancer?

Many people who've been through a cancer experience, particularly one that requires long-term treatments, say that some relationships are intensified and others fall away. You'll find out who your real friends are and you'll discover that special people come into your life for the duration of your intensive treatments. These can be nurses, hospital acquaintances, or casual acquaintances who have a special feeling or

understanding of your current problems. The most complex
changes in relationships usually occur within the family.
There is an opportunity for growth and greater intimacy, or
the possibility of greater misunderstandings. Friends can be
a major source of support, or, if they have trouble dealing
with their own anxieties, may start avoiding or rejecting you,
often not returning until what *they perceive* as the threat of
death has passed.

What is the most difficult time for cancer patients?

In a study by the California Division of the American Cancer
Society, which surveyed the needs of 800 patients and more
than 100 family members, it was shown that 30 percent of
patients said the key stress period was just after the diagnosis; 16 percent felt it was the period of hospitalization and
initial treatment; and 11 percent felt that the most stressful
time was the period after release from the hospital. Many
patients found it very difficult to share their feelings about
their illness with either family or friends. Some coped well
with stress initially, but experienced delayed reactions six or
more months later. Depression may continue, often for prolonged periods, even after successful treatment. Where and
how to find help during this period of time is discussed later
in this chapter.

**Why do I have a feeling of numbness about my whole expe-
rience?**

Sometimes this feeling can last for weeks. It is an emotional
state that serves to detach you from your feelings and allows
you to deal with your problem with your mind rather than
with your emotions. Very often, learning you have cancer is
such an emotional blow that it blocks out your ability to face
your future. Everything is put on "hold" and you go through
the motions of your treatments without really thinking about
what is happening.

Why do I feel as though my body has let me down?

Many people are plagued by this same feeling. It's probably because you have worked hard at strengthening your body, eating nourishing foods, taking good care of yourself. When your body develops cancer, it's as if all your caring was useless. You feel a loss of control. Your sense of your own mortality is heightened. But don't despair. You can use these feelings to examine what is most important to your life. Start taking control by being a partner with your doctor in making decisions about your illness and its treatment. And remember that a body that's in good shape will continue to cooperate in the healing process.

Is there any evidence that knowing the details of what is going to happen to me during and after treatment helps me get better faster?

A study was done at Massachusetts General Hospital on patients who were going to have abdominal surgery. One half of the patients were told in detail about the kind of pain they might have after the operation, where it would occur, how long it would last, and how painful it would be. This group was also told that this pain was normal and they were taught how to relax to ease the pain. The other group of patients were not given any special information. The result was that the people who were told the details of what would happen asked for half as many painkillers and narcotics as did the other patients. They were also able to leave the hospital three days earlier on average than did the uninformed group. If you are not given written information or if the members of the treatment team have not spent time with you and your family to explain what to expect, ask that this be done. You might take a tape recorder with you so that you will have something to refer back to and to share with other family members.

Is it a good idea for me to try to humanize my stay in the hospital?

It can be difficult, but as soon as you feel up to it, you can start wearing your own clothes, keeping yourself as well groomed as you do at home, conducting yourself with the positive attitude of someone who knows he/she is going to get well—and quickly. It's wonderful for your morale. Paintings and photographs that have meaning, your own special pillow, green plants and flowers, all help to make you feel more at home and in control. Special treats—if diet permits—milk shakes from the corner drug store, a hot pastrami on rye, or some other coveted goodie help make life more bearable. The important thing to keep in mind is to let everyone know, in a polite way, that you expect to be treated like a special human being rather than as a hospital fixture.

Is it true that laughter is physically good for you?

Laughter has physical benefits. A good laugh gives a workout to several parts of your body. It relaxes your diaphragm, your lungs are exercised, your body's oxygen level increases, many of the muscles in your face, chest, and stomach are activated, your pulse rate and blood pressure may go down. Relaxation and anxiety cannot exist together, so, since laughter relaxes your body, your anxieties decrease. There are some studies which show that laughter also stimulates some brain chemicals which may help lessen pain. Norman Cousins, in pain with a rare, supposedly fatal disease, made a practice of watching humorous videotapes and felt that his hearty laughter played a big role in his recovery. His book, *Anatomy of an Illness* (Norton, 1979), tells about his personal experiences with serious illness and how positive emotions and the patient/physician partnership cured him. Humor can take your mind off your troubles and make you feel better. A videotape machine is a good investment. You can rent videotapes and give yourself the gift of a good old-fashioned belly laugh.

"I laugh more and cry more. I give more hugs and compliments. I don't put off things. I keep very busy trying to live a whole lifetime in the next few years."

Diagnosed with lymphoma in 1984 at age 38

Is it a good idea to get back to normal routine as quickly as possible?

Routine can operate as a healing force. The act of getting your life back to normal becomes therapeutic. The routine involved produces greater strength. Looking forward to a task, even when you're uncertain whether you are up to it, helps give you the stamina to do what needs to be done. Find things to look forward to—simple things like being with your friends at work, going out for an ice cream cone, going out to dinner, or being able to resume some household or work-related task.

Why is it that some days I feel wonderful and other days I'm ready to give up hope?

Everyone agrees that living with cancer can be like living in an elevator. The trauma of the treatments can sometimes cloud the vision and make even the most optimistic person feel like giving up. The interplay of life and death is never more vivid than when we are in the midst of such a medical crisis. What is most needed when depression hits is someone to talk with, someone with whom you can share your true feelings, someone who can give you moral support. Psychologists tell us that there are two kinds of hope: passive and active. Passive hope is the fairy-tale kind where we dream of miracles. People with active hope use their strength and imagination to make miracles come true. There is hope in the fact that cancer obeys no laws. You may find it helpful to write down exactly why you feel you are ready to give up hope. Study your reasons. Try to outline positive ways of acting on your loss of hope to guide you when you lose your hopeful feelings.

Why do I spend so much time worrying?

Worrying is part of the work of the mind that is a natural response to danger. Naturally, you perceive cancer as a danger and threat to your life even though you know you will probably be cured. Worry is your mind responding to such danger. Worry can be compared to the work of grieving or mourning. It can be therapeutic. The times around diagnosis, treatment, and checkups are critical worry times. Waiting for any of the interminable treatments in doctors' waiting rooms, X-ray rooms, or therapy centers heightens your worry. Worrying is a normal part of acceptance of what has happened to you. You can learn to channel it into a positive force.

Is it normal for me to get angry as a result of worrying?

Getting angry is one of the ways people cope with worrying. When you are diagnosed with cancer, feelings of disbelief and uncertainty can last for days, weeks, and months. The situation is highly stressful, so don't be surprised if you experience major mood swings, depressed one day, irritable the next, agreeable on another day. Some of these changes can be due to medications—so it's important to know what medications are being given and what the side effects are. Someone who lashes out at family members may actually be expressing anger toward the disease or desperately trying to disguise a deep-felt fear. Most people enter this personal crisis time using whatever their coping mechanism has been for other major problems—possibly in a more exaggerated way.

Does a fighting spirit really help to improve chances of a cancer cure?

A great deal has been written on this, but a recent study of 57 women followed for 10 years after they were diagnosed with breast cancer sheds some light on the subject. It was found that women who stoically accepted their diagnosis had the highest death rate and those who met the diagnosis with a fighting spirit had the lowest. The way in which people face their problems certainly seems to make a difference. One woman deliberately took charge by announcing that she was assembling a team to take care of her. She interviewed surgeons and plastic surgeons, and invited her friend, an oncology nurse, to join her "team." Taking control is one way of dealing with the situation in a positive way. Taking control also means expressing negative emotions like anger, anxiety, fear, and depression. Stress levels are usually highest in the three months after the diagnosis—and it often takes six months to a year to work through all the emotions that the disease can stir up.

Is it true that the right kind of anger helps you to come to grips with cancer?

Several studies indicate that patients who get angry at the fact that they have cancer are most likely to live longer. Of course, the kind of anger you vent is also an important factor. One kind of anger is petty and destructive—it leads to aggressive and destructive behavior—and includes lashing out at those around you for no good reason. The other sort of anger is justifiable anger, the kind that is directed against a disease you cannot control. Expressing anger at having cancer is a necessary stage in coming to grips with cancer. It may be difficult to experience this anger without feeling shame or guilt. Because many cancer patients feel that they need the support of others in order to survive, they are often reluctant to express anger openly and end up being compliant and turning the anger inward to themselves. Don't deny yourself the expression of honest anger. The inability to experience it leads to lowered physical resistance and symptoms of depression. Practice getting in touch with your deepest feelings. It will give you a sense of personal authority.

Is the will to live important?

The will to live is the ability to harness a great deal of your personal energy—encouraging and aiding the body to do its own natural healing. Through the ages, healers and doctors have known that some people are able to overcome illnesses while others, often less ill, get worse and die. Modern scientists have been trying to unravel the mysteries of why this happens—and have tried to determine how spontaneous remissions, for example, are related to the consciousness and psychology of the person who is cured. The elusive will to live can be strengthened through a powerful technique known as self-hypnosis. These forceful energies, which are not fully understood, can be controlled and directed by individuals to bring about healing.

Will the underlying feeling of being afraid and despairing ever completely leave me?

Fear and despair, anxiety and depression, are all natural emotions that will come and go. As you put more time behind your treatments, these emotions should decrease. Gaining control over your health care, understanding what is natural and normal in the course of your illness and what is not, expressing your anger about your illness, admitting your fears, all will help you to regain control over your life. The most important thing you can do is to learn all the facts about your illness. Since each case is so different from any other, it is important for you to understand the nature of the type of cancer you have.

Is it important for me to understand what the side effects of my treatments are?

It is really important for you to know all about the possible side effects to lift the burden of unnecessary worry. Some patients mistakenly interpret the usual side effects—such as nausea, appetite loss, tiredness, itching—as signs their cancer is getting worse, when actually what is happening is a normal reaction to treatment.

How can I keep up my spirits when treatments are so long-term?

Techniques for helping yourself to get through treatments that stretch over a long period of time include:
- Setting some long-term goals for yourself. Allowing yourself to look forward to some event in the future—a vacation, a short trip, or a special occasion such as a wedding or graduation. Making plans for the future helps the future arrive faster.
- Not allowing your life to get so bogged down that treatments are the *only* thing you have to look forward to. Plan a lunch date with a good friend, arrange to see the latest movie, keep up your interest in your favorite team. Don't hesitate to make plans for a long-dreamed-of vacation. Discuss your plans with your doctor. Getting the cooperation of your doctor and having something positive to think about will make you feel better.

Am I wrong in being hopeful about my health even though my doctor continues to give me negative feelings about how I'm doing?

This is a case where you need to question your doctor to find out what he means by the signals he is giving to you. It may be helpful for you to seek an opinion from another doctor. You may decide at this point that you need to change doctors. It's important to have a doctor who understands the way you think—someone who is encouraging rather than discouraging, who can give you legitimate reasons for hope. If you are not getting this kind of positive feedback, you need to think through why you are staying with this particular doctor. In addition, you should do your own homework, learn about your specific kind of cancer, so you can ask questions and have enough background to understand the progress and limitations of your present status.

"The emotional recovery took longer than the physical. Talking about it helped me heal emotionally."

Diagnosed with early cervical cancer in 1987 at age 27

Why do some doctors who treat cancer patients seem distant and unfeeling?

The doctor/patient relationship in cancer treatment is very intense. As a result, unlike doctors in other specialties who can complete treatment by writing a prescription, the oncologist must see the patient through a series of treatments and often attempts to put emotional distance between himself and his patients. Many patients find, however, that breaking down the barrier by being open with the doctor, asking to be a partner with him in making decisions, and being honest with him about feelings is the best way to bring about a change in his attitude.

Why should I stick with a treatment that is difficult?

Such treatments, like chemotherapy or radiation, in most cases, are set up so that you know, generally, when they will begin and when they will be completed. If you skip out on treatments, you're cutting yourself off from the full benefits. You'll increase your chances of being cured if you can keep your sights on the future and stay with the treatments, even though they may be difficult and debilitating. Down the road, you know when they are going to end. Counting down the treatments, treating yourself to extra days off from work at the critical times, being especially good to yourself, can all be helpful in making it easier for you to deal with the present.

Is there psychiatric help available for cancer patients who are having trouble facing their illness?

There are a number of ways to deal with getting help in facing your illness. Some people find that a few one-to-one sessions with a mental-health professional are helpful in making them feel more comfortable with changes in their bodies, as well as giving them skills for coping with cancer. Others find that support groups or individual sessions with hospital or community social workers are helpful. Across the country there are also some highly specialized people who deal with "situational" crisis. If you feel the need, you can ask the doctor or the hospital social worker for a referral to someone who deals in crisis intervention. A nonprofit institution in Westchester County, New York, called the Situational Crisis Service of the Center for Preventive Psychiatry, for example, is staffed with clinical psychologists who deal with situational crisis intervention. These professionals are trained to give ready understanding and practical direction to indi-

viduals and families. There is a great deal of professional help
that can be given so that the situation can be dealt with in an
unfrightened, upbeat, positive way. Help is given to the entire family. Patients and family members are taught how to
deal with anger, jealousy, resentment, and guilt. They are
allowed to verbalize feelings. Priorities are reordered and
options are exercised.

What kind of support groups are available?

There are two kinds of support groups available—support
groups led by health professionals, and self-help groups
which are run by people who have cancer. Both types of
groups offer encouragement, information, strategies for coping, and a wonderful place to form friendships with others
who understand your problems.

What groups are available through the American Cancer Society?

The national American Cancer Society provides local units
with resource materials for setting up a variety of support
groups. Many mutual support programs that began as
grassroots efforts have been designated as national programs
of the American Cancer Society. CanSurmount brings together the patient, the family member, a CanSurmount volunteer, and a health professional. Upon referral from your
physician, a trained CanSurmount volunteer, who is also a
cancer patient, meets with the patient and family in the hospital or home. The I Can Cope program addresses the educational and psychological needs of people with cancer and
their families. A series of eight classes meet to discuss the
disease, how to cope with daily health problems, how to express feelings, living with limitations and local resources.
Through lectures, group discussions, and study assignments,
the I Can Cope program helps people with cancer regain a

sense of control over their lives. The Reach to Recovery program is designed for women who have had breast cancer. Volunteers—women who have already adjusted successfully to their mastectomies—visit new patients, both before the operation and after surgery. Chapter 9 contains information on support groups.

How do self-help groups work?

Sometimes, despite the fact that we have the most sophisticated professionals responsible for our care, there is a real need to get beyond the technical knowledge and talk over our situations and problems with other people who've had the same experience. Self-help groups are often administered by hospitals, the American Cancer Society, or other organized groups, or can be the simple outgrowth of a group of people who share the same problems and want to help one another. Many members of self-help groups find they move from being helpees to becoming helpers, from students to teachers, from dependent learners to independent doers. Knowledge is traded and shared. Practical advice is exchanged and everyone benefits.

How can I find out about self-help groups in my area?

You can check with your doctor, the social services department in your hospital, or make a call to the American Cancer Society in your area. You can find the number in the White Pages of the telephone directory. The American Cancer Society is a good source of information about what's available. Groups are sometimes listed in the Yellow Pages under Social Service Organizations or Health Agencies. One organization that has a long history in the self-help area is Make Today Count. The address is 101½ South Union Street, Alexandria, VA 22314-3348; telephone: 703-548-9674. A newer group is the Wellness Community, founded by Harold

Benjamin, who hopes to establish a nationwide network. This group is operating in two locations in California and has branches in Massachusetts as well. It offers free group therapy with licensed psychotherapists, plus freewheeling discussion sessions that include the trading of life stories, encouragement, and the use of directed visualization. In many communities, groups belonging to the National Coalition for Cancer Survivorship (323 Eighth Street, SW, Alburqurque, NM 81102) run self-help programs. There is more information on self-help groups in Chapter 9.

Can I start my own self-help group?

If there are no self-help groups in your area, it is possible to get one started on your own. Many health professionals—nurses and social workers primarily—have had training in starting groups. Basically, the steps in getting a group going include:

- Get in touch with other self-help groups for ideas on how they are organized. Many groups are based on the Alcoholic Anonymous model. Others are set up on a much looser basis.
- Form a core group of two or three interested people. Decide how the group will operate and how planning will be shared.
- Seek out a professional—nurse or social worker—who is willing to serve as a consultant. This usually means helping the group to become organized, providing advice and counsel, but not assuming responsibility for actual leadership, decision making, or group tasks.
- Plans for meeting times and place and organization development should be agreed upon. Time should be allowed for all members to introduce needs they feel the group might address. At the close of the first meeting there should be a general consensus on the needs of the group and agreement on a suitable site and time for the next meeting.

- The group will need to consider whether meetings will include guest speakers, films, or special service projects as part of the educational program for members, or whether it will be strictly a discussion group. Many groups establish audiotape libraries, lending libraries of informative books and medical articles, etc.
- The organizational structure may be as formal or as informal as members prefer—with or without elected officials and written bylaws. A professional advisory committee may be helpful.
- Groups vary enormously in their style and manner of functioning. Conflict and disagreement are a normal part of any group. However, it should be established that the goal is to listen, explore options, and express feelings. Try to stay away from prescribing, diagnosing, judging, or giving advice. An important rule to be established is to actively listen when someone is talking and avoid having side conversations or interrupting.
- The first phase of the group's life should be devoted to letting people get to know each other and enjoy each other so you can start to build the group process. It's important not to go too fast but to build traditions slowly and carefully.

What are the benefits of a self-help group?

There are many benefits that we have seen from self-help groups. The most important is getting to know other people with similar problems and observing how they deal with them. Further benefits include developing networks of help, helping others, developing coping strategies, getting feedback from others, acquiring a feeling of control over problems, and receiving the rewards of a strong support system.

Questions to Ask Yourself

- Am I doing everything I can to understand my kind of cancer?
- Do I feel a need to change doctors?
- Am I ready to contact or start a support or helping group?
- Should I change the direction of my life by changing jobs or lifestyle?
- Can I start a candid discussion with my mate, a special friend, or my children about my feelings?
- Is thinking about cancer overtaking my life and can I start changing that by doing one of the above?

ACTION: Pick one and resolve to do something about it NOW.

chapter 2

Getting Your Life Back to Normal

Life turns upside down when you're dealing with cancer. Everything is disrupted. Doctor appointments and hospital visits seem to take over your life. Everything you do revolves around your treatments and your health. People rally to your side. Cards and flowers, gifts and telephone calls, occupy your time. But the day quickly arrives when you know you must concentrate on normalcy. The adjustment back to living a normal life, though it sounds strange, can be a major one. To your own surprise and confusion, the joy and release you'd anticipated may not be quite as you expected. During convalescence and treatment you feel protected, involved in the fight to save your life. When it's over, there is often a feeling of vulnerability. It's a normal reaction—so don't let it panic you.

Your main task will be to focus on getting your life back to normal as soon as possible. You'll need to work to build a high level of wellness, through a healthy lifestyle, stress management, proper diet, and exercise. But before you can get on with normal living, you may have to deal with some emotional baggage that comes with having cancer.

Why is it so hard for me to concentrate on what I'm doing?

Your anxieties can create mental disorganization, confusion, and memory disturbances, and give you a feeling of being constantly distracted. Sometimes you may experience a general feeling of loss of motivation. Even simple tasks like writing a check, dealing with routine business tasks, cooking a meal, filing insurance bills, or making necessary phone calls can seem overwhelming. Once you concentrate on the fact that you're feeling overwhelmed because of your underlying health concerns, you can begin to focus your energies on calming yourself and getting past your distractions. You'll find that the passage of time helps to put your anxieties into perspective.

How can I deal with the constant uncertainty that goes with having cancer?

While some cancers are cured following surgery and treatment, there remain ongoing, long-term, unbalancing concerns that can give you a feeling you are not in control. Many people cope with this by keeping very accurate and complete records about their case, continuing to follow research and new therapies available for their type of cancer. Many maintain that when they face up to uncertainty by doing something positive and constructive, they gain a feeling of control as well as a feeling of hopefulness.

How do you deal with the post-convalescence letdown and jar yourself back into action?

The time immediately following the end of treatments can be difficult because it is a cut-off point without the focus of the routine that had occupied you following diagnosis. This may increase your worrying and anxiety levels. Getting back to work, to school, and/or to your normal routines as quickly as possible is important. Taking up some new hobby, starting a new class, getting involved in something that allows you to absorb yourself completely are good ways to force yourself back to feeling alive again. The numbness gradually disappears as you invest yourself in living.

"I let my friends and family help me, spend time with me, read to me, remind me of the beauties of the world. A nurse encouraged me to make strawberry jam one day when I wanted only to lie in bed. I found that I felt weak getting up—but no weaker than I did when I lay down. I'm so glad she pushed me."

Diagnosed with lymphoma in 1984 at age 38

How can I cope with all the stress I feel?

Having cancer is stressful. Learning to cope with that stress requires knowledge of yourself so that you can take steps to control it. Admitting your stress, recognizing the tenseness it brings, is the first part of conquering it. Keeping as occupied as possible, stepping up your exercise, going for a walk, giving yourself permission to enjoy yourself are all steps that help you to cope with the stress you feel.

What are some ways of keeping occupied when I cannot pursue my normal routine?

- Encourage telephone calls and chatting on the phone. Ask friends to call on a rotating basis.
- Painting, drawing, and sculpting with clay are wonderful pastimes, even for someone who hasn't worked with art supplies before.
- Pets are a wonderful distraction. Fish tanks are soothing and absorbing to watch. Kittens, dogs, and birds are fun.

- Absorbing TV and video programs—such as light enter-
tainment, tennis, baseball, and football matches, educational classics, and old movies—can be a welcome
distraction.
- Computer games require little physical strength and are a
wonderful way to pass time.
- Tape recorders are tremendously useful for recording letters to family and friends as well as for listening purposes.
Many books are available on tape and some libraries carry
a selection of both books and music on tape.

---

*"My new puppy, who gave me unconditional
love, really helped in my recovery. That, and the
love and caring of my family and friends."*

*Segmental left breast surgery and lymph node
surgery, 1984, at age 41, followed by
chemotherapy and radiation*

**Are there ways to make myself feel better when I'm feeling
down?**

A study which looked at how people manage to comfort
themselves in difficult times may be helpful. The research,
headed by Paul Horton, a psychiatrist in Connecticut, surveyed 160 men and women from the ages of 22 to 74 and
ranked the 10 most popular sources of solace. These included: being with someone else, listening to music, watching TV, eating, reading, talking to oneself, prayer, reading a
special book such as the Bible, recalling pleasant memories,
and going for a walk—all simple and doable pursuits.

Why is it so hard for me to solve my own problems?

People often have trouble being as compassionate or rational
about their own problems as they are with other's problems.

Psychologists suggest that you try writing down your thoughts and feelings. In one column list your thoughts and fears. In the next column write a rational response to each thought. When it's written down, it's easier to see when you are distorting things—imagining the worst thing that could happen or being too harsh on yourself. Some people find that actually talking aloud to themselves, as opposed to a silent, internal dialogue, gives a better sense of perspective. It may be helpful to ask yourself what you would tell a friend in a similar situation.

What kind of problems do most people who have cancer experience?

Family problems seem to be common in at least a third of those surveyed. Such problems as change in behavior of children in the family, fear of dying, anger caused by the diagnosis, financial burdens, sexual difficulties, a feeling of neglect by the partner, drinking, gambling, frequent absences of the partner, and fear of giving the disease to others, were all mentioned by patients.

How does cancer change people's daily lives?

Most often there is a change in the way roles are handled within the family. If someone in the family is hospitalized frequently or for a long time, or has physical or psychological effects with cancer, he or she may not be able to fulfill the usual role. The problems involved in redistributing these roles depend on the stage of the family in the family life cycle, the communications patterns within the family, and the family's way of dealing with change. Some of the most common changes involve the following roles, which can be disrupted by even the most subtle changes: financial provider, household organizer, child carer, child socializer, sexual partner, maintainer of family relationships, hand-holder, family social life organizer. Most family members have roles that come to them because of age or sex, characteristics over which they have no control. Beyond that, most have roles that are achieved through the member's own efforts and abilities. With changes forced upon the family by hospitalization and treatment, roles are disrupted, the family's cohesiveness decreases, family conflict can increase, and until roles are realigned, strains upon the family begin to show. Some family members will take on greater burdens with the reassigned roles and will feel overloaded, and as a result, problems can occur. Being aware of these possibilities can help to relieve the strains put upon everyone during these times.

What kind of changes can be made to help relieve strains?

The healthy family members can help to redistribute some of the load. Help can come from outside the family, from parents and grandparents, brothers and sisters, neighbors and friends, or through people hired to help during the crisis. Greatest disruptions naturally occur in families where there are young children. A study done at Ohio State University shows that when the nuclear family is relied upon to assume some of the reassigned roles, there is less conflict than when outside help is used. It's best, if at all possible, to encourage children to continue sports and after-school activities. If the family has a tradition of going to the movies every Friday night, for example, try to get back to that routine as soon as possible.

Are my feelings that I have less energy and tire more easily due to my cancer treatment or am I just imagining that?

Many people report that they feel their energy level takes a long time to return to normal—often a year or two after treatment. Studies have also shown that some people are still struggling with problems of tiredness two or three years after

treatment has ended. There is strong evidence that exercise
can be helpful in combating these side effects.

What kind of exercise can I safely do?

Choose a way of exercising that is something you enjoy. Do it
until you are relaxed and pleasantly tired. Don't turn it into
another stress in your life. Walking is one of the best ways to
exercise. Many people are taking advantage of indoor shopping malls for comfortable, weather-free walking. Some malls
are even opening early to encourage mall-walkers. There are
many advantages in using a mall for walking. It is heated in
winter and cooled in summer. You don't have to worry about
traffic or whether or not you are safe. The surface you walk
on is smoother—no ruts or holes. All you need is a comfortable pair of shoes. Any kind of repetitive exercise, such as
walking, running, swimming, rowing, gives you a chance to
relax, meditate, or visualize, because you don't have to think
about what you are doing. You can pay attention to what your
body is saying as you exercise.

**What other forms of exercise/relaxation can I be consider-
ing?**

Relaxation means different things to different people. However, most people fall into one of three categories: physical,
mental, or mixed. People who are physical feel tension in the
body. They get the jitters, the "sweats," or diarrhea. Mental
types experience stress mainly in the mind—worrying, or
with mind-blocking thoughts. Mixed types usually have an
equal amount of physical and mental stresses. Physical people might consider these possible relaxation methods: aero-
bics, swimming, bicycle riding, rowing, walking, yoga,
massage, sauna or soaking in the hot tub or Jacuzzi. Mental
types find that the sheer exertion of physical exercise does
not work, but that engaging the mind and redirecting it is

helpful. Meditation, mental relaxation techniques, reading, crossword puzzles, jigsaw puzzles, movies or TV watching, chess or card games, TV games, and crafts such as knitting, carpentry, and so on, may be helpful. Mixed types often find that a physical activity that also demands mental exertion is relaxing. Competitive sports such as tennis, racquetball, or volleyball, meditation, or any combination from the physical and mental lists may prove to be right for them. You may wish to try some new activity that will make you feel good about yourself. Just be careful not to push yourself too hard, especially while you are in treatment.

"During treatment, be positive, but get your emotions out. If you're having a bad day, give yourself the okay to complain about it, but realize that the reason you're having a bad day is so that you'll have better days.

"Do things that make you happy—hobbies, people you like to see, theater, trips. Don't dwell on the fact of being ill."

Ovarian cancer, stage II, 1979, at age 29

Do meditation and exercise go hand in hand?

The effects of meditation are multiplied when combined with exercise. Meditation also has physical effects on the body. Like exercise, it tends to lower blood pressure and pulse rates. Brain-wave patterns change, showing less excitement. The blood has fewer stress hormones in it. There are some studies that show a connection between meditation and the immune system response.

Is there something I can do to lessen my stress?

People who've been through the cancer experience say that it helps to be very kind to yourself. Think positively about who and what you are. Think through the things you are really interested in doing and do them. Many people never find time to do the things that mean the most to them because they spend so much time doing things that are meaningless to them. Try to find something that you enjoy that relaxes you. Some people find walking, sailing, tennis or golf especially relaxing. For others it could be square dancing or fishing. Think through what's important and fun for you that will lessen the stress you put on yourself. You may find that promising yourself "rewards" at different times during treatment—such as going out to dinner when you've finished a cycle of chemo—can help to lessen stress and make positive progress. Look for occasions to treat yourself in extra-special ways.

Is rehabilitation help available for cancer patients?

Until about 10 years ago, most rehabilitation services were prescribed for persons with physical handicaps. Recently, rehabilitation efforts have been extended to patients with cancer and heart disease. Nearly all cancer patients can benefit from rehabilitation services. The focus is on physical, social, psychological, and vocational needs. Reach to Recovery (a rehabilitation program for breast cancer patients), International Association of Laryngectomees, United Ostomy Association, Candlelighters, and the I Can Cope programs are all support groups that have been formed to help the cancer patient return to normal living. About 30 percent of patients need assistance with activities involved in daily living and in coping with pain. About 15 percent are deeply concerned about their physical appearance. Arm or leg swelling or breathing problems are of concern to about 10 percent, and about 7 percent have needs in communication and transportation. Many have multiple difficulties that need attention. Try to find the services that will help you deal with your particular needs and help you to live normally.

What kinds of help can you expect to get from a rehabilitation team or physiatrist?

Depending on the severity of the situation, the team members will vary but the goal is to help you to readapt and to live as normal and full a life as possible. In some cases, a physiatrist—a doctor who specializes in rehabilitation techniques, including the strengthening of muscles, the use of artificial limbs, and retraining in day-to-day activities—may be required. Physical therapists or occupational therapists often work together to teach patients the skills needed to allow them to perform their daily tasks. In the case of a mastectomy patient, the physical and occupational therapists sometimes work together to teach arm exercises that will help overcome swelling and weakness to allow the patient to continue her daily life without discomfort. Oncology nurses are often helpful in assisting the family to help the patient become more independent and can help in planning at-home care and rehabilitation. They are skilled in helping deal with the many psycho-social issues involved with cancer. Social workers, members of the clergy, and lay volunteers can be called upon to provide assistance and advice in both religious and personal matters. Psychologists and other mental-health professionals, speech pathologists, dieticians, pharmacists, all can play a part in helping you to readjust.

How do you know who to call for help?

Though help is available, it can only come to you with your consent and at your request. Many people suffer needlessly because they are afraid to ask for the help they need. Many are reluctant to discuss problems such as changes in sexual or body functioning or in appearance, and thereby shut off the possibilities of getting help. It is important to discuss any of your needs frankly with your physicians, nurses, or the social workers at the hospital where you were treated. Home health-care agencies and services such as the American Cancer Society, Visiting Nurses, and public health departments are helpful in pinpointing the specific services that can be utilized over a period of time to assist you. Most of them can be reached with a simple phone call, and most of them are more than willing to help you determine what help you need and who is best to call to obtain that help.

Must my employer take me back as soon as I am ready to go back to work, even if I will be taking time off for treatments?

The answer depends upon what kind of employment you have and what federal and state laws cover it. It is best to talk with the benefits department in your company to find out what the policy is. Ask your doctor or nurse to help you figure out how you can combine work time with your treatment time. There may be a way for you to arrange for treatment late in the afternoon or on weekends so that you can continue working with little time off. You might need a referral to an occupational or a physical therapist to prepare you to return to work. You should discuss your employment situation with your doctor so that, if necessary, he can talk with your employer's benefits or medical department.

Are most people able to return to work after having cancer?

It is encouraging to know that at least 80 percent—the vast majority of people with cancer—go back to their former jobs without problems. Several studies have found that these returning workers have turnover rates, absenteeism, and work performance comparable to all other employees. There is also a study which shows that recovered employees were better than average because they felt compelled to work harder to prove their wellness.

What kind of problems do recovered patients have to face in the workplace?

There are still some employers and employees who carry the old groundless fears, including the belief that cancer may be contagious or that the patient will somehow affect fellow workers. Some employers assume that cancer patients will continue to require time away from the job. Facts and studies show that this is simply not true. Recovered cancer patients often have better work records than those who have not had cancer. Nonetheless, 54 percent of recovered patients say that they had problems at work that they felt were a result of their illness. Some of the problems discussed included: hostility of fellow workers, lack of salary advances, reduced health benefits, exclusion from life or disability insurance, and reluctance to use sick leave even when justified. Many reported difficulties in finding new positions and an increase in the cost of insurance premiums.

Why do some people resort to lying about having had cancer?

Because of the stubborn stigma that cancer still carries in the minds of some people—including some employers and coworkers—some cancer patients who have recovered and returned to work say they have resorted to lying about their disease. One friend, who had a bone cancer in the shoulder removed and was left with difficulty in shoulder movement, said that she changed her story and began telling people who asked that she had been in a skiing accident. She reports that people treated her differently after she changed her story and that she was no longer passed over for promotions.

How honest should I be in filling out an application for a new job?

You can be honest without disclosing your entire health history. You should be aware that your employer needs to know your health history only as it affects your ability to do the job for which you are applying. Moreover, that knowledge is needed only after you have been given serious consideration as an applicant. While most cancer patients go back to their jobs, 20 percent report that they have been subjected to discrimination. Among reported problems are: not being able to get a new job, losing a job or being transferred from present positions, being demoted or not promoted, or having duties taken away. Young people, especially those who have never been employed before, have the highest rates of being denied new job opportunities. Employers claim that fear of higher health insurance rates is the main reason for being wary about hiring those who have had cancer. Insurers say that small companies—which is where most jobs are—fear that their group health insurance may be canceled if they hire someone with a history of cancer.

What can I tell an employer during a job interview when I'm asked about my health?

You can answer that you want the job and that you intend to be a faithful, hardworking employee. If you have had an attendance record at your last job that reflects the fact that you were absent because of your cancer experience, you can stress your attendance average in terms of how many days per month you have been absent over the entire period of your last employment. You can stress how productive you are and voice your determination to be productive if you get this job. Phrases like "I like to work and I give my best to every job I've ever done" can help present you in a positive way and change the focus of the question.

Why do employers still discriminate against people who've had cancer?

Mostly they discriminate because of their own fears and lack of information about cancer. They say they are hesitant to invest in an employee who, in their minds, may die. They consider their judgments to be business ones—citing fears that insurance companies will increase their rates or refuse to insure them. They fear that the employee will become less and less productive because of medical problems. In fact, half of all individuals in the United States diagnosed with cancer this year will overcome the disease. For those under age 55, survival rates are even higher. Decades of studies confirm that cancer survivors have the same productivity rates as other workers. Millions of individuals remain as productive or more productive after a cancer diagnosis than they were before.

How does the law protect a healthy, able-bodied individual with a history of cancer who is wrongfully perceived by an employer as being unemployable?

Although no comprehensive federal cancer survivor bill of rights has been written, national lawmakers have expressed their outrage at discrimination based on cancer history, and some laws for the physically handicapped have been cited in cancer discrimination cases. In June 1986, the National Conference of Mayors adopted a resolution prohibiting discrimination against cancer patients. In September 1986, the United States House and Senate unanimously passed House Concurrent Resolution 321 expressing opposition to cancer-based employment discrimination.

Federal and many state laws provide protection for those who are termed physically handicapped—a stereotype most cancer patients feel does not apply to them. Be that as it may, the laws which protect those who have had cancer from employment discrimination are most often contained in provisions protecting the physically handicapped.

The major piece of federal legislation is the Rehabilitation Act of 1973. Section 503 of the Rehabilitation Act generally covers employers who have contracts or subcontracts with the federal government. Section 504 of the federal law applies to "programs or activities" which receive federal financial assistance. Federal employers are also governed by the Rehabilitation Act.

Physical handicap is defined as "any person who (i) has a physical or mental impairment which substantially limits one or more of such person's major life activities (ii) has a record of such an impairment or (iii) is regarded as having such an impairment." Regulations which implement Section 503 underscore these rights. The regulations read: "'Has a record of such an impairment' means that an individual may be completely recovered from a previous physical or mental impairment. It is included because the attitude of employers, supervisors and co-workers toward that previous impairment may result in an individual experiencing difficulty in securing, retaining, or advancing in employment. The mentally restored, those who have had heart attacks or cancer often experience such difficulty." Unfortunately, while the federal law has a very broad definition of "handicapped," it applies to only a limited number of employers. If an employer is not governed by the federal Rehabilitation Act, you must turn to state laws for protection. Forty-five states and the District of Columbia have laws that prohibit employment discrimination against the physically handicapped by both private and public sector employers. Legal protections vary from state to state, and must be addressed on that level.

The American Cancer Society and the National Coalition for Cancer Survivorship are taking leadership roles in organizing to stimulate the national conscience on behalf of those who are faced with discrimination because of cancer.

Are most co-workers supportive of a person with cancer?

Attitudes vary. Some studies have found that co-workers can
be among the strongest support networks. However, blue-
collar workers were less supportive than white-collar
workers. Those people who had cancers that were most easily visible, such as on the face or neck, had more problems
with co-workers than did those whose cancer was not as easily seen. People who had long absences, took off many extra
days, or were tired and weak and thus not able to complete
their work as before had more work-related problems. On
the other hand, in the study of white-collar workers, it was
found that co-workers willingly took on extra duties and gave
moral support and encouragement to cancer patients.

Is it true that I may be denied life insurance because I have had cancer?

Many people with a cancer history are able to get life insurance. It may be necessary to pay a higher price. If the cancer
is a major one and recently diagnosed and treated, you may
have to wait a few years before you are fully eligible. Life
insurance premiums are based on how many people who are
healthy at the time they buy insurance will live a given period of time. If you have a serious disease when applying for
insurance, you either pay a higher premium or the insurance
may be denied. Most companies look carefully at the site,
type, grade, and stage of cancer when evaluating an application. If you do not get a favorable response from the first
insurance company you try, ask your insurance agent to refer
your application to a life insurance broker who will know
which company is likely to make a fair review of your history.
(Brokers belong to an association called the National Association of Life Brokerage Agencies.)

Some companies have special programs for cancer and for
other chronically ill patients. The insurance may not be at

the lowest rates, but at least your application will get a realistic review. A few companies have a "graded benefit policy" in which only premiums paid are returned if the insured person dies within the first few years. After three or four years, the full face amount of the policy goes into effect.

If I leave my job, can I still be covered by group life insurance?

If you are covered by group life insurance where you have worked and it was a major company, it may be possible for you to continue to carry the group life insurance policy on your own. In most states, the insurance company must offer people who leave their jobs for any reason individual life insurance without any health requirements at a premium for the age. If you are lucky enough to be working for a large company, some life insurance may be available to you under these provisions. Smaller companies may have insurance policies that do not allow this kind of transfer coverage.

What kinds of insurance are easiest for recovered cancer patients to be eligible for?

Group insurance is probably the best option available for recovered cancer patients. Because there is no legal requirement that an insurer grant coverage to anyone, and because, legally, insurance companies can set premiums at any level, provided they are based on sound actuarial practices, independent insurance coverage can be a problem for people who have had cancer.

The Rehabilitation Act of 1973 specifically lists those with a history of cancer under the federal definition of the disabled. Employers who receive federal funds must provide equal fringe benefits, including insurance, to disabled individuals as they do to other employees. These employers are prohibited from discriminating in terms of hiring or promotion and cannot ask questions about an employee's health unless the questions are specifically job-related. Noninsurability cannot be used as a reason to deny employment. Certain employers receiving federal funds also must take affirmative action to ensure that disabled persons receive equal employment. Prepaid health plans and health-maintenance organizations that meet federal requirements are forbidden by federal law from canceling services. In addition, they must provide an annual period of open enrollment when coverage is offered on the same basis as it is to all other members. It is illegal to charge higher premiums to those who might require increased usage.

What are the best ways of getting insurance if you have a cancer history?

You need to explore every possibility if you are not already insured or if you have had changes in your present insurance. Here are some suggestions:

- Check to see if such plans as Blue Cross/Blue Shield have an open enrollment period. During open enrollment, you can join regardless of your health history.
- Try to get group insurance through an association such as a professional group (teachers, accountants, artists, trade or fraternal groups).
- If you have a chance to work for a large company, take it. Most large companies offer group insurance that gives benefits to all employees regardless of health history.
- If you are permanently disabled and have been getting Social Security benefits for two years, or if you are 62 or older, you need to investigate whether you are eligible for Medicare. You also need to look into a supplemental policy to Medicare which covers the costs it will not cover. If you are unemployed or have a low income, you may be eligible for state assistance such as Medicaid.
- If you have served with the military, look into possible veteran's benefits.
- Check your insurance conversion benefits before you change jobs or leave a job.

- The federal law (Consolidated Omnibus Budget Reconciliation Act of 1986—COBRA) requires that companies with more than 20 employees allow employees leaving a job to extend medical benefits for up to 18 months. Both employees and surviving, divorced, or separated spouses and dependent children are covered by this provision. This applies if you are leaving a job, working fewer hours, have quit, or are fired. You must be certain to make arrangements for extension with your personnel office before you leave.
- Contact an independent broker who may be able to help you find a benefit package at a reasonable rate.

Where can I turn if all my health insurance benefits are used up?

About one fourth of the states have some form of health insurance pool for those who are uninsurable. The first such pool was established in Connecticut in 1975; because of this arrangement, insurance in the state is available to all. Under the Connecticut law, the losses incurred by the insurance companies are shared by all—the commercial insurers, Blue Cross/Blue Shield, HMOs, and self-insured employers—on a pro rata basis. Insurance pools in some states have waiting periods; that is, if you come into the plan with a cancer history, you would not be reimbursed for claims arising out of any treatment for cancer for the first six months (or 12 months, depending on the plan) of participation in the plan. However, you would be covered for other health costs not related to cancer during that time.

What should I do if my insurance company turns down some of my claims?

Even the most standardized policy provisions are subject to widely different interpretations from company to company. If you have a complaint, or feel that you have been treated unfairly by your insurance company, agent, or broker, be sure to report it to your state insurance department. Also, send a copy of your letter to your state representative or senator.

Control Your Attitude

You're in control of your attitude.
The way you think makes a difference in how you feel.
You have a choice of being negative or positive.
You can turn negative happenings into positive ones by how you view things.
Focus on the positive aspects of what's happening to you.
Positive attitudes make for positive results.
With a positive attitude you are in control.
No matter what happens, you can deal with it.

---

chapter 3

The Healing Mind

Many people who have conquered cancer believe that by using their own spiritual, mental, and emotional resources—natural skills which every human being possesses—they have been able to create a strong, new state of health within themselves.

The idea that mind and body are both somehow responsible for health and disease is certainly not new. As long ago as the fifth century B.C., Greek physicians taught that whatever happens in the mind influences the body, and whatever happens in the body influences the mind. The latest research is indicating that the most significant factor in maintaining good health may be a sense of control over events in life. A person's ability to control how he looks at demanding or difficult situations, and how he reacts to them, can be reflected in his health. A variety of basic techniques are being used by many cancer patients to enhance their feelings of well-being, to reduce stress, and to promote relaxation.

Some of the more common techniques include:
- Relaxation
- Hypnosis
- Visualization
- Prayer
- Biofeedback
- Verbal therapy
- Healing guides
- Psychic healing

Can people really influence their cancers through attitude, psychological interventions, or lifestyle?

This question will be debated for a long time. Medical science has not come to any firm conclusions. Many people feel uncomfortable with the so-called voodoo approach. However, new technological and scientific developments such as the new imaging devices, which help researchers see precise images of brain activity, are making it easier for scientists to explain the effects of psychological and social factors. The body fights off disease by taking advantage of the immune system. Research has established that stress and its consequent activity in the brain can directly affect the work of these immune cells. Many people feel that they have been able to have influence over their emotional response to cancer, with great impact on their personal quality of life. Whether or not the biology of the disease is influenced remains an individual and open question. Some have said that they feel a sense of failure or guilt when the disease progressed after they had tried some of the various self-help methods. Others maintain that the sense of control gained by using these methods is important to their well-being and point out that they do not have time to wait for scientifically proven results.

"I had good examples in my family—especially my aunt who has survived two mastectomies and has been cancer-free for at least 10 years. Two of my aunts had breast cancer, three of my sisters did, too. My mother was a victim of late-discovery breast cancer. I went back to work right away and kept on with my life. I prayed a lot and laughed a lot."

Stage II breast cancer, mastectomy, chemotherapy

What can I do if my doctor doesn't believe in the self-help methods of healing?

Discuss your thinking with your doctor. You'll probably be surprised at how supportive he will be in your efforts to use your mind to help you in healing. As long as he understands that you will continue to be cooperative in following his prescribed treatments, there is no harm in experimenting with some of the self-help methods. Healing happens in your own body. Your doctor can help you to heal. Your doctor is highly skilled and intensively trained in the mechanics of how your body works. He's seen many people with the same cancer problems. But treatments are only part of the picture. Since your aim is to be healed, don't hesitate to draw from whatever resources are available and seem to make sense to you.

What is the basis for mind-control techniques?

The movement is an extension of Buddhist and Hindu practices used by Orientals for several thousand years. Tens of thousands of Americans and Europeans adopted the basics of these practices in transcendental meditation, popularly known as TM, as a means for developing human potential. From this movement came the great variety of mind-control methods that have become a part of American life and have been taken up by the medical and scientific community for pain control and healing help. Mind control embraces the entire field of biofeedback, relaxation, visualization, and meditation, each using its own techniques to expand the mind and allow the body to enter a new dimension.

In this chapter we seek only to sketch the basic information needed for you to begin to try the various methods to see if they appeal to you. The techniques involve a creative growth process, not a rigid or formal therapy, and you must discover it by yourself. Many who try complain that at first they find the experience confusing and frustrating. Once

they learn to concentrate, with awareness deliberately controlled, attention is directed and relaxation takes over to
allow the mind to do its work. For those who are interested
in delving deeper, there are many books and videotapes that
deal with the subject.

How do I use relaxation?

Learning relaxation techniques can be very helpful to you in
allowing you to let go of your stress. It is the basis for many
of the other techniques you may want to employ in using
self-help in healing. There are many different ways in which
you can learn to relax. A number of commercially available
tape recordings provide step-by-step instructions in relaxation techniques. There are several simple methods that you
can learn quickly:

- Inhale/tense, exhale/relax. Breathe in deeply. At the same
  time, tense all your muscles or a group of muscles of your
  choice. For example, you can squeeze your eyes shut,
  frown, clench your teeth, make a fist, stiffen your arms
  and legs, or draw up your arms and legs as tightly as you
  can. Hold your breath and keep your muscles tense for a
  second or two. Let go. Breathe out and let your body go
  limp. Relax.
- Slow rhythmic breathing. Stare at an object, or close your
  eyes and concentrate on your breathing or on a peaceful
  scene. Take a slow, deep breath and, as you breathe in,
  tense your muscles (such as your arms). As you breathe
  out, relax and feel the tension draining. Now, remain relaxed and begin breathing slowly and comfortably, concentrating on your breathing, taking about six to nine
  breaths a minute. Do not breathe too deeply. To maintain
  a slow, even rhythm as you breathe out, you can say silently to yourself, "IN, one, two; OUT, one, two." If you
  feel out of breath, take a deep breath and then continue
  the slow-breathing exercise. Each time you breathe out,
  feel yourself relaxing and going limp. If you feel that some
  muscles are not relaxed, tense them as you breathe in and

relax them as you breathe out. Continue slow, rhythmic breathing for a few seconds up to 10 minutes depending on your need. To end, count silently and slowly to 3. Open your eyes. Say silently to yourself: "I feel alert and relaxed."

Why is it so hard for me to get myself into a relaxed state?

Learning to relax yourself completely may be hard at first. Practice the simple forms of relaxation several times during the day. You may try doing relaxation exercises sitting up or lying down. Try to choose a quiet spot. Close your eyes. Do not cross your arms and legs because that may cut off circulation and cause numbness or tingling. If you are lying down, be sure you are comfortable. Put a small pillow under your neck and under your knees, as well, if you find that comfortable.

Is there a quick relaxation theme that's been found to be most universally helpful?

One that is most commonly mentioned as being helpful is the beach scene. Think of your favorite beach spot. Recall the pleasant warmth of the sun and the tranquilizing sound of the waves. Imagine yourself basking in the warmth and let the sound of the waves lull you into relaxation. Always try putting yourself inside the scene, rather than being on the outside looking in.

What is imagery and how does it work?

Imagery means using your imagination to create mental pictures of situations. It can be thought of as a deliberate daydream that uses all of your senses—sight, touch, hearing, smell, and taste. Some believe that imagery is a form of self-hypnosis.

What's a quick technique for trying out how imagery works?

First, close your eyes. Breathe slowly and allow yourself to feel relaxed.

Do this for a few minutes. Then imagine a ball of healing energy forming in your lungs or on your chest. You might imagine it as a white light. Imagine it forming, taking shape. When you are ready, imagine that the air you breathe in blows this healing ball of energy to the area where you have cancer, where it heals and relaxes you. When you breathe out, imagine the air blows the ball away from your body, taking the cancer cells with it. Continue to breathe in, bringing the ball of energy to the spot, and breathe out as the ball of energy takes the cancer cells away. To end this exercise, count slowly to 3, breathe in deeply, open your eyes, and silently say to yourself: "I feel alert and relaxed."

"To keep a positive attitude I used mental imagery, visualization, and I prayed. I belonged to a cancer support group which gave me courage. Our support leader made a personalized tape which I listened to, especially when I could not sleep at night. I listened over and over until I fell back to sleep."

Diagnosed with inoperable lung cancer in 1984 at age 46, now in remission after radiation and chemotherapy treatments

---

What is visualization?

Visualization is a technique in which the mind is given a strong mental experience that it almost cannot distinguish from an actual physical experience. It has been used in a variety of ways over the last few decades. Carl and Stephanie Simonton adopted some of the techniques used by Silva

Mind Control after learning that users of biofeedback often were able to communicate with their bodies more effectively by means of an image than by directly trying to influence a certain organ or function. Dr. Bernie S. Siegel has used a similar method with his patients. His book *Love, Medicine & Miracles* (Harper & Row, 1986) explores the link between mind and body, and lists techniques and tapes available to aid patients in influencing their own recoveries.

How does visualization work?

No one understands precisely how it works, but psychologist Charles Garfield studied cancer patients who recovered at the University of California Medical Center in San Francisco and concluded that most of them had the ability to enter states of mind that enabled their bodies to perform at extraordinary levels—much as trained athletes do. Garfield found similarities between their behavior and the behavior of athletes who had used visualization techniques originated by the Bulgarians for use with their Olympic teams. These same techniques are being used by most super-athletes in the United States and in countries all over the world. It is possible that visualization takes advantage of the way the mind works—using a strong mental image that cannot be distinguished by the mind from something that actually happens.

How is visualization and imagery being used in other fields?

The sports field has been using the concept of visualization and imagery for many years. Jack Nicklaus is well known for promoting its use to achieve better athletic performance. Several Olympic stars, including diver Greg Louganis, high jumper Dwight Stones, and runner Mary Decker, practice visualization before they compete. Russian researchers, in studying the effects of goal setting, relaxation, and visualization on world-class athletes, found that those who spent three quarters of their lives in strong mental training and one quarter in physical training showed significantly greater improvement. In teaching visualization for sports use, concentration is focused on specific movements. It is believed this creates neural patterns in the brain so that the more often you visualize the movement, the more ingrained the patterns become. Thus, when the brain tells the muscles how to move, these patterns are called upon and used. NASA research has determined that it is possible to imprint on the brain an image of a physical event before it happens, making it easier for the person when he or she actually performs the action.

How are sports figures taught visualization?

Most are taught to visualize in a step-by-step process. First they are instructed to write down the entire process in three different ways—they write about preparing to compete, about the actual competition, and about their action and feelings when they win. Goals are set for each part, focusing on what the person wants to achieve and the end result. The athletes are told to describe as vividly as possible the details of each phase of their participation—the excitement of being part of the event, the crowds, the weather, the sounds and smells. The written description includes feelings of being in control of their physical and mental state, imagining relaxation, and detailing smooth performance at each point in the match or event. Next, they are taught how to review their written material, looking for flaws and making changes until it satisfies them. They are then instructed in relaxation techniques and in the use of visualization of what they have written. This step-by-step process allows the athletes to make the program a part of themselves, feeling it, seeing it in written form, and internalizing it.

How does visualization work for athletes when they are performing?

Some say they actually see the movements and all that goes along with them in their minds. Others say they "see" only through strong feelings in their bodies, while still others may hear only the sounds or the rhythms. However, in rigorous athletic training, visualization tries to use all the senses, concentrating them in the brain to foster confidence and achievement. Many do a final visualization before they go to sleep, and the next day "play the film back" as they get ready to compete.

Is the use of visualization and mental imagery growing in cancer treatment?

More people are using visualization and imagery in combination with other treatments for cancer. As a matter of fact, the use of the mind to foster good health in general is a growing field, including teaching relaxation techniques and the use of hypnosis.

How can I make visualization work for me?

The first step is to learn the art of relaxation. Then you can start perfecting the mental picture that addresses your problem in your own way. You can imagine your brain turning off the valve that directs the flow of blood to your tumor. Some people picture the cancer cells as crabs. One person said he could imagine a fisherman scooping them up in the net. Another pictured the crabs shriveling up and disappearing. You might choose to think in more medical terms—of your white cells attacking cancer cells and destroying them. If you are on chemotherapy, you can imagine the drug as coming in and zapping off the cancer cells. Or, you might think of your white cells as white knights or rocket ships battling and killing off the cancer cells. The important point, in visualization, is to learn to focus your attention on directing your body to do something positive about changing your cancer situation. Many patients are making a point of spending some quiet time each day facilitating the healing process by concentrating on the healing energy in their bodies.

I have a hard time getting myself relaxed enough to do visualization. Are there any techniques for making it easier?

Some people find, when they first start, it is difficult to learn the techniques and reach relaxation. You may find it helpful to use a tape recorder, with a relaxation tape you've bought or made yourself. Making your own tape can be helpful. You may want to enlist the aid of a friend to help you investigate the technique. It's important, in making your own tape, to go at your own speed. Give yourself images that you enjoy, talking slowly and in a relaxed manner. Leave yourself time on the tape to enjoy each stage. Though some experts feel it is better to learn to be free of the tape, if it works for you, this is a good way of teaching yourself the techniques so they become a part of you. If you feel you wish to open your eyes, tell yourself first that you are relaxed and it will be hard to open your eyes. Then, open them, see the room you are actually in, close them again, and practice returning to the relaxed state. Repeated use of the technique will make the images more and more vivid. You can do this several times, each time telling yourself that you'll be even more relaxed when you close your eyes again. Use the tape recorder as long as you feel comfortable with it. Once you've learned the techniques, you may find that the tape is confining and that you can be more creative and relaxed without it. Relaxation becomes easier each time you practice.

Where can I find more information on relaxation and visualization?

There are many books on the subject. *Relaxation Response* by Herbert Benson (G.K. Hall, 1976), *Love, Medicine & Miracles* by Bernie S. Siegel, M.D. (Harper & Row, 1986), *Getting Well Again* by O. Carl and Stephanie Simonton (Bantam Books, 1982), and *How to Meditate* by Larry LaShan (Boston: Little, Brown, 1974) are some that you may find helpful.

Can I use visualization techniques for stopping nausea?

Concentrating on relaxation has been found to divert the body's attention away from the negative. Triumphers have told us that positive thoughts work best. Rather than thinking, "My nausea will stop," which negatively focuses on the nausea, they suggest, "This is going to make me thirsty and hungry," or "I'm going to be famished when this is over."

How are pictures or drawings done by the patient used to change attitudes of cancer patients?

This technique was first used successfully with children with leukemia who were unable to express their fears and concerns. It was found to be so helpful that it was adopted for use with adults. Many therapists are now using the technique—learning to interpret drawings so that conflicts can be identified. Then, work is done to resolve the conflicts, and often visualization techniques are used to reprogram the unconscious. Dr. Bernie Siegel explains the technique and shows some of the drawings in his *Love, Medicine & Miracles*. He asks patients to draw themselves, their treatment, their disease, and their white cells eliminating the disease.

He also asks for at least one drawing of a scene. In addition, his patients are sometimes asked to draw themselves at work, at home with the family, in the operating room, or wherever he feels there are areas of conflict in the person's life.

Dr. Siegel explains that the most common conflict is in the patient's attitude toward treatment. The patient often says, "I know this treatment is good for me," but unconsciously feels, "This stuff is poison." He works with patients to change the attitude through visualization—making the patient conscious on an intellectual level that this is what may be blocking his progress. He feels that the drawings are a way to get people to open up and talk about things they would otherwise conceal, even from themselves.

What is verbal therapy?

Verbal therapy is the use of words and voice to affect changes. We've all talked to ourselves at one time or another —and we all know that talking to ourselves is a way of preparing ourselves mentally, physically, and emotionally for some event. We tell ourselves to slow down or hurry up. We admonish ourselves to calm down when we're about to lose our temper. We all do it, and we do it because it works. You can do it deliberately by talking to your whole self, or you can concentrate on a specific part of your body. Think of your mind and body as a computer that needs positive commands given to it. One helpful exercise calls for programming a statement which represents what you wish to happen, such as "I feel better and better every day." Take a few minutes to repeat it over and over, imagining how good you will feel and the positive results of the improvement. Do this whenever you have a few spare minutes—while waiting in a line, driving to work, stuck in a traffic jam, folding the laundry. Get into the habit of verbally giving yourself positive suggestions when talking with others as well. Listen to how you answer when people ask how you are doing. Do you describe yourself as sick, weak, tired? These words can act as self-suggestion, which can react internally.

How are "healing guides" used to visualize?

This sounds way out, but it is being used by some people who claim it is a powerful technique. Some people refer to the technique as "healing angels" or "imaginary doctors." Here's one way to go about using it: Visualize a comfortable space, such as an office or library, well furnished and inviting. Imagine an automatic button marked "Health Adviser" or "Healer." In your relaxed state, push the button and watch the door open. Someone will enter. This will be your healing guide. You can start asking questions about your condition and listen to the answers. You may want to write down what you hear. If you're not happy with the guide or with what you are told, you can release that guide from duty and push the button and try again. After all, this is your imagination working, and you can summon up whomever you wish in any way you wish. If no one seems to come through the door, you can construct your guide based on your ideal of what you would like the guide to be. Visualize your healer in your environment sitting down to talk. Perfected over time, this scenario can become another way of training your mind to help you deal with your body.

How is therapeutic touch used in healing?

Everyone has the latent ability to use his own natural energy in healing. The technique is being taught at many nursing schools across the country. Scientifically, it is believed that electron-transfer resonance explains what happens when hands are used to transfer energy to another part of the body. Some people unconsciously are able to focus their natural bioenergy field and become known as healers. But everyone can learn to do it and it is possible to use the basic technique on yourself:

- Start by taking three deep breaths to relax your muscles.
- Rub your hands together in a circular, clockwise motion for 15 to 30 seconds.
- Hold your palms six inches to a foot apart for a few seconds and imagine there is an energy field between them, growing stronger and stronger.
- Cup your fingers inward, place your hands just above the area to be treated, and imagine the energy entering the area and healing. It may help to imagine the energy as a bright color.
- Rub your hands again and reapply.

Is the idea of going to a psychic healer absolutely crazy?

We know lots of perfectly sane people who have gone to psychic healers and have found help and comfort in doing so. Your doctor, and other people too, may think you have lost your mind or gone around the bend, but our experience with people who have been through a cancer experience and tried using a psychic healer indicates that psychic healing is another tool that can be used to good advantage if it interests you. Psychic healers share with others their supply of bioenergy to aid the healing process. Naturally, you are wise to use this type of healing to supplement any other type of healing you are practicing rather than as a substitute for the type of treatment you are receiving from doctors. If you are afraid to try a psychic healer, then you should probably forget about it, because fear may inhibit possible healing benefits.

How does biofeedback work?

The basic concept of biofeedback is quite simple. Biofeedback uses electronic signals to teach you how to master the control of your body's automatic functions, such as heartbeat, blood pressure, and muscle tension. The electronic machinery is wired to you and your involuntary functions are monitored and reported through light or sound signals. Through observation of the results, you learn to regulate your body. In learning how to relax muscles, for example, patients are wired to a machine that picks up the electrical current produced by a muscle when it contracts. The machine converts this signal to a light or sound. The person learns how to turn off the signal by relaxing the muscle. With practice, muscle relaxation can then become a conscious action. Biofeedback means getting immediate, ongoing information about one's own biological processes or conditions. Biofeedback training means using the information to change or control voluntarily the specific response being monitored.

Can you do biofeedback on your own?

Biofeedback is best taught with professional supervision. If you want to continue biofeedback on your own, once you have learned how, several home devices are available for under $100. The most common is the digital thermometer, which may be purchased with sensors that attach to the body. It should have a continuous readout and be sensitive to differences of 0.1 degrees. Another device measures galvanic skin response (GSR), which measures the perspiration on your skin. Because you perspire more when you're tense, GSR is a widely used measure of tension. Wristwatches that continuously read out pulse rate can also be used. Biofeedback is a tool. You train your body to achieve the relaxation results that the device is measuring. The device serves as a graphic demonstration that you can regulate your hand temperature or your pulse rate. To locate those people in your area working on biofeedback, look under Biofeedback in your local telephone directory.

Can hypnosis be used in healing?

The American Medical Association approved hypnosis as a tool back in 1957 and it is being taught to medical students as a technique in medical school. The greatest therapeutic tool we possess is our mind. Many of us think of stage hypnosis when we hear the word—where an otherwise inhibited, reserved person completely changes character and does wild, crazy, unthinkable things. Most hypnotists say this is not the case, that if people are given a suggestion they don't want to obey, they do not follow it or they simply come out of hypnosis. But the power of suggestion has tremendous force and it has been found that about 60 percent of the population can be hypnotized.

How can I find a qualified person for hypnosis?

Your local medical center may be able to provide you with referrals. Many medical centers are using hypnosis for treatment of pain. You might consult a doctor, a psychologist, or a hospital-affiliated social worker who has experience with hypnosis rather than going to someone who is simply billed as a hypnotist. There are many unqualified people who practice hypnotism. The county medical society or one of the following organizations may be of help in locating a qualified hypnotist: The Society for Clinical and Experimental Hypnosis, 128A Kings Park Drive, Liverpool, NY 13090, or The American Society of Clinical Hypnosis, 2250 E. Devon Avenue, Suite 336, Des Plaines, IL 60018, 312-297-3317.

How do I practice self-hypnosis?

There are many different ways of achieving a self-hypnotic state and there are numerous books that cover these methods. Most people start out by going to a qualified hypnotist before they try it on their own. We will outline one basic way in which you can achieve a state of relaxation to induce self-hypnosis.

STAGE ONE: Sit comfortably with your feet on the floor or lie down on a couch or mat. You can direct yourself to relax, or you can repeat a prayer or phrase, fix your eyes on one spot or object, or listen to a monotonous sound, such as the ticking of a clock or dripping water. Any of these can be used to prepare you so you are ready to progress to the next stage. Once you feel ready to relax fully through one of these methods, close your eyes, breathe deeply, and feel your muscles becoming loose, limp, and relaxed.

STAGE TWO: Some people can become profoundly relaxed with one of the Stage 1 self-hypnosis methods. For most people, however, a second stage of relaxation is necessary to go deeper. You can use any or several of these methods to help you sink into deep relaxation:

- Deep-breathing method. Start breathing deeply, counting slowly from 1 to 10, feeling yourself becoming more and more relaxed. Suggest to yourself that by the time you reach 10, you'll be in a state of deep relaxation.

- Staircase or elevator method. Imagine yourself standing barefooted at the top of a beautiful staircase or in a plushly lined elevator that leads down, down, down. The stairs are covered with a thick, luxurious carpet that gets thicker and more luxurious as you go down the stairs. You begin thinking of yourself walking down the carpeted steps, one step at a time, moving slowly. Each step down makes you feel more and more relaxed. Suspended above the stairs as you descend are numbers, from 1 to 5. As you pass each number, you feel more and more relaxed and you know that when you reach number 5, you will feel completely relaxed.

STAGE THREE: Now you are ready to take yourself into the third stage. Imagine a comfortable space that is your very own. It is furnished to your own taste—whatever environment you feel relaxed in. It could be a beautiful room, a lovely garden, a spot by a babbling brook. Make it a safe, neutral spot where you can pause and luxuriate. After experiencing the quiet for a few moments, find a place where you can sit or lie down. Now you can begin to focus on your visualization—seeing your treatment and your immune system removing cancer cells from your body. Try to form active pictures of how this happens. Tell yourself how wonderful you will feel, how well you will be as the cancer disappears from your body. When you feel ready, you can gradually begin to return from your hideaway, walking to the stairs, climbing the stairway upward, passing level five, then four, then three, then two, and finally one. Take some deep breaths—each breath making you feel better and more alert. Realize that when you open your eyes, you'll feel wonderful and refreshed.

After doing these exercises several times a day, you'll be able to do them more quickly and easily each time. No two people do them in exactly the same way, but it can be satisfying and productive.

Can meditation be helpful?

Meditation, like relaxation and self-hypnosis techniques, is another way of disengaging your mind from everyday thoughts and focusing it in a different direction.

What is a mantra and how is it used?

A mantra is a word or phrase that one repeats over and over again, until it becomes internalized instead of spoken. It is used in meditation, in yoga or Hindu practices, though it has also been used by other philosophical and religious systems. "One" or "Om" or "Peace" or "I am relaxed" are frequently used. Some medical studies have shown that the practice of repeating a word over and over can release stress and produce certain health benefits by inducing a generalized state of physical relaxation. To try this technique, sit comfortably and find some word, syllable, or phrase that you enjoy saying over and over to yourself, letting the mind focus naturally and as effortlessly as possible on the mantra.

What are some of the kinds of healing phrases that others have found helpful?

Here are some we have learned from triumphers:
- I am relaxed and comfortable.
- I am calm and serene.
- I am one with the earth, sun, and stars.
- I can feel myself being bathed in God's healing light.
- I am peaceful.
- I feel strong.
- My mind and body function perfectly and normally.
- My immune system protects me from cancer cells.
- My body knows how to heal itself.
- I am becoming healthier and healthier.
- I am free of illness, pain, and worry.
- I feel only love.

Do many people find their religious beliefs helpful in coping with cancer?

Most patients we have talked with have told us of the help they received from their religious beliefs. Several studies have shown that most people call upon their religious beliefs to help them through their cancer crisis. A study of 50 patients at the University of Alabama Comprehensive Cancer Center found that 80 percent felt their religious beliefs helped them in coping with their cancer. This same study also noted that half felt the overall quality of their lives was better after cancer than before their diagnosis. They worried less about material things, they appreciated friends and families more, and their religious beliefs became clearer. These people were realistic yet hopeful, and were combining this hope with renewed interest in their daily lives and involvement with people.

Have You Had These Feelings?

rage
anger
anguish
helplessness
shock
fear
disbelief
numbness
resentment
confusion
guilt
panic
apathy
crying spells
listlessness
depression
self-pity
dread
worry
hostility
fear

They're all perfectly normal. It would be unusual NOT to have some or all of these feelings. It's perfectly okay to have them—but now it's time to do something about them.

Charting Your Feelings, Fears, and Beliefs

TRUE   FALSE

_____ _____ I like to know everything that is happening to me.

_____ _____ I want just the barest details about my cancer.

_____ _____ I need to get more information about what's happening to me.

_____ _____ Information about cancer is too painful to grasp.

_____ _____ My doctor is not telling me enough.

_____ _____ I want my doctor to be absolutely frank with me.

_____ _____ I want to be able to discuss my fears, anxiety, and discomfort.

_____ _____ Knowing I will not be abandoned adds to my sense of comfort.

_____ _____ I hope everyone will understand my continuing need for concern.

_____ _____ I prefer a businesslike approach from my doctor.

_____ _____ I want my doctor to be warm and empathetic.

_____ _____ I want my doctor to be aware of the way I live my life so he can understand how that affects my treatment.

_____ _____ I want one doctor to be my primary source of information.

_____ _____ I find it hard to deal with so many doctors.

_____ _____ I am not able to talk with my family about my fears.

_____ _____ People treat me as though I'm dying.

TRUE	FALSE	
_____	_____	I don't want to be pitied.
_____	_____	I have accepted my new life circumstances and will master this situation.
_____	_____	It is distressing to have people who know nothing about my cancer try to diagnose and offer suggestions.
_____	_____	I have a new awareness of death and how precious life is.
_____	_____	I'm scared.
_____	_____	My family and friends are overprotective.
_____	_____	I hate false cheerfulness.
_____	_____	I'm angry at having cancer.
_____	_____	I'm afraid I may die.
_____	_____	I'm lucky to have such good doctors.
_____	_____	I will be completely well again.
_____	_____	I could have prevented cancer if I'd lived differently.
_____	_____	My attitude will affect my quality of life.
_____	_____	I hate having cancer.
_____	_____	I can think myself ill.
_____	_____	I can make my body stronger.
_____	_____	I'm embarrassed by my fears.
_____	_____	My cancer can be controlled, if not cured.
_____	_____	I can tell people I have cancer.
_____	_____	My cancer is a long-term proposition that I will learn to live with.
_____	_____	I want to share my fears and concerns.
_____	_____	My anger isn't against my family, just against what's happening to me.

TRUE   FALSE

_____ _____ I'm afraid of being left physically and psychologically alone.

_____ _____ I'm not depressed.

_____ _____ I feel at peace with myself.

Take stock of your answers. Go back and mark those you intend to do something about. Write them out on 5 × 7 file cards. Make plans to start taking action on those that make you feel in control.

Put Your Goals in Writing

Write each of these goals, or any others that fit your thinking, on a 3 × 5 file card and review them often.

I'll be positive.

I feel better.

I will avoid people and situations that make me feel negative.

I'll use visualization to change the things I'm unhappy about.

I'll allow myself time to just enjoy.

I'll be good to myself because I'm a very important person.

I'll appreciate what others do for me and let them know it.

I'll remember that nothing in life stays the same.

I'll welcome new experiences so that I can continue to change as my world changes.

I'll let go of my anger.

I won't take myself or my problems too seriously.

I'll look for humor-cherishing, witty, funny, beautiful moments.

I'll be honest with myself and others.

I'll spend each day living, not dying.

I'll work at being a good communicator so others know where I stand.

I'll try to relax to make me feel better.

Dealing With Problems

- What problems do I see this illness creating?
- How am I going to deal with them?
- How do I usually deal with problems I must do something about?
- Who do I usually turn to for help?
- What kinds of problems usually get me down?

Making yourself aware of your behavior patterns will help you to concentrate on dealing with day-to-day experiences positively.

Facts to Remember in Using Relaxation Techniques

TRY all the different relaxation and visualization techniques, then use the one that suits you best on a regular basis, once or twice a day for five or 10 minutes at a time until it becomes easy and routine. You should not use these techniques for more than one hour a day.

REMEMBER that your ability to use relaxation techniques may vary from day to day.

DON'T try to force relaxation. If you have a problem using a technique, use a quick and easy method like breathing in and tensing and breathing out and relaxing.

TRY NOT TO cross your arms and legs. Change your position if you feel tingling or prickling in your arms and legs.

DO take a deep breath if you have a sensation of shortness of breath or of suffocation. Sometimes, however, this feeling may be caused by breathing too deeply. If this is the problem, take shallower breaths and breathe more slowly.

IF the technique puts you to sleep and you don't want to go to sleep, try sitting in a hard chair. You can also set a timer or alarm as insurance.

chapter 4

What Happens to Sex?

Sex sometimes takes a back seat when you have cancer. Sexual functions you took for granted—feeling the wonderful sensations of pleasure, having an erection or an orgasm—often stop functioning under situations of pressure, tension, and fear. Sometimes this causes partners to withdraw emotionally. Sometimes, previous sexual patterns must be altered because of body changes. In the sexual area, most of us do not verbally communicate very well. So even the smallest change can result in tremendous problems. Each of us, young or old, healthy or ill, regardless of marital status or sexual preference, has a deep need to be loved and cared for and to have someone with whom to share that love. This delicate relationship is often upset when you have cancer. All the stresses and strains that go with cancer diagnosis and treatment often disrupt the balance of relationships.

Learning to discuss feelings and talking about intimate needs with those close to you can help you and those you love to understand and accept the changes in your life. Many studies have shown that communicating your feelings to others is necessary to physical, mental, and emotional well-being. For individuals with cancer, their partners, families, and friends, it is doubly important, because cancer and treatment can affect how you feel about yourself in so many ways. Your body has changed, and this can affect you both physically and psychologically. You may need help in understanding the changes, what they are doing to you and how you can start to deal with them. You may be experiencing a range of emotions—feelings of vulnerability, of depression, of anger. You may have problems in achieving intimacy because of changes in your body image or because of real, imagined, or anticipated feelings of rejection. Some of the normal reactions after illness—of trying to do more than you should be doing, or overcompensating for having been sick—can be blocking your normal reactions. Treatment may be affecting your sexuality, either as a direct side effect or by dulling your response to touch so that timing is thrown off, making it take longer for you to respond. You probably have found that you have more of a need to maintain closeness, to have that special bond and focused relationship with your partner. Understanding what your needs are and sharing your new understanding will help to make your sexual encounters more pleasurable.

Are most sexual problems following cancer likely to be permanent?

The answer depends, of course, on the treatments you have had to cure your cancer. Most problems, however, are of a temporary nature. Once healing is complete and treatments are over, and the stress and fear have subsided, you'll feel more relaxed and ready to enjoy sex again. Many doctors and patients are often hesitant in talking about the effects of cancer treatment on sexuality. Find out from your doctor what the expected effects are on sexuality for the type of cancer treatment you are receiving. When you know what to expect, you can plan how you will deal with those problems. There are a number of questions you may wish to ask your doctor:

- Will my ability to have sexual intercourse be changed temporarily or permanently?
- When can I have intercourse again?
- Will the operation or treatment leave me sterile?

- Will my treatments affect my ability to have an erection/climax?
- What changes should I be on the lookout for?
- What are the sexual side effects of treatment? Are they temporary? How long will they last?
- Are there any other kinds of treatments I could consider?
- What are the benefits and risks of those treatments?

Don't be embarrassed to ask questions about this very important part of your life. Make a list, and be sure to ask for details if the answers are not clear. Knowing what to expect makes it easier to deal with the changes. Just as important as talking frankly with your doctor is discussing what you learn with your partner and others who love you, so that they understand what is happening to you.

"The man I had been with for six years was sure I would not be as sexual as I had been before the operation. Was he surprised! There was no change at all once healing was completed."

Hysterectomy for cancer of endometrium, 1983, at age 66

Why is it that I have little or no sex drive since I found out I have cancer, yet I need a lot more hugging and reassurance?

The way you feel is quite normal and can be expected to change as you become less stressed. Lack of sex drive can happen during many different stages of the disease—at diagnosis, at various times during treatment, when new treatments need to be undertaken, or when you feel ill. At these times, there is a great need for physical contact, though not necessarily for sexual intercourse. Partners should be aware that the special warmth of a loving touch conveys feelings in a very direct way. Sitting or lying together, holding each other, cuddling, holding hands, kissing, a warm hug, gentle stroking of the hair, or a relaxing back rub are all ways of being sexual and fulfilling the need to be physically close. You need to let your partner know how important it is to you to continue be touched and held even if you do not want to have intercourse. *Your partner is waiting for cues from you.*

Will having intercourse harm my incision?

This is an important question to ask your doctor. In the early days after an operation, it is important not to put unnecessary strain on the incision. During healing, sexual intercourse may cause bleeding or may strain the incision. Intimate contact at that time may also increase chances of an infection. The time between surgery and resumption of sexual activity varies, but once the healing is complete and your doctor has assured you that you may resume normal activities, you should try not to worry about hurting yourself. Be careful not to use the operation as an excuse to postpone sex, when other reasons are really at the base of your lack of desire. Be honest with yourself. If it is not simply that your scar is tender, but that you are embarrassed or depressed about your scar or that you fear that your partner will be put off by the operation, then it will be helpful if the two of you can talk about this.

Should I take special precautions to avoid infection?

During treatment, and for a time after treatment, when your immune system has been weakened, you may be vulnerable to infections. You should take special care to avoid sexually transmitted diseases. Genital herpes, gonorrhea, and AIDS viruses are especially dangerous when your immune system is under stress. So it is important to be careful in choosing partners. You can reduce your chances of exposing yourself to these diseases if the man wears a condom or the woman uses a vaginal contraceptive such as foam, a diaphragm with jelly or cream, or one of the new vaginal sponges.

How can I approach my partner about resuming sex?

Many people react to cancer by withdrawing into themselves. They are afraid to share their feelings of fear and loss. They are reluctant to expose themselves to possible rejection. The result is that both partners are left to deal with their individual kinds of loneliness. If your partner acts in a distant manner, you become more and more reluctant to make a sexual advance because you are afraid of appearing demanding and unfeeling. Try to discuss your feelings openly—not in a demanding or accusing fashion but in a positive way ("I miss having sex so much. Let's talk about why it's become a problem for us and how we can have fun experimenting").

What happens if we are unable to resume normal sex?

The most important ingredient in helping you to enjoyment is communication. Learn how to talk with each other about your needs. Your sexual routine will need to change, but it can still be pleasurable. Let your partner know, either in words or touch, what feels best for you. The most important thing to remember is that no matter what the health circumstances, there is absolutely no reason to give up the warm and wonderful closeness that being together and touching can bring.

Can masturbation be helpful?

One way to begin to determine your own capacity to enjoy sex again is to start with self-stimulation. If your religious, social, and cultural background permits, masturbation is a form of sexual activity that can be satisfactory when sexual intercourse is not possible or desired. Some women have found that mechanical vibrators can be helpful, either for self-stimulation or along with other sexual activities with their partners.

Why does my loss of weight following cancer surgery make me feel so sexually unattractive?

Loss of weight and the weakness that goes along with it can take a toll on your feelings about yourself. Even though the old adage says you can't be too thin or too rich, sudden weight loss can be very depressing. Changes in your body, which weight loss seems to emphasize, can sometimes make you feel that your sexuality is threatened.

Why does my loss of appetite cause relationship problems with my partner?

This is a common question. When attention becomes focused on your diet, other areas of your relationship seem to be affected, too. In our society, where food is used to express care and love, the reaction when you are unable to eat is likely to be one of disappointment and rejection. In turn, you may feel guilty because you aren't hungry and your partner went to a great deal of trouble to prepare food for you. It's important for you both to understand the many emotions behind the eating questions so you can work together to resolve them.

Will my interest in sex ever return?

It depends upon what is causing your lack of interest. If it is caused by your feelings brought on by having cancer and treatment, it will probably be temporary and decrease as time goes on. If it is caused by the medications you are taking, it will probably disappear when you go off the medication. If there is a physical cause for the problem, the question needs to be discussed with your doctor. Often cancer patients must become accustomed to the changes in their bodies and the way their bodies function. Hair loss, weight change, or surgery, for example, may cause embarrassment and make it difficult for you even to think about being involved in a sexual relationship. Sometimes these feelings take quite a bit of time to sort out and understand. Although surviving cancer may bring you closer to those you love, it is not unusual for it to temporarily affect your sexuality. If, after a reasonable period of time, your interest does not return, you should seek the help of a professional.

Why is it so hard to talk to my doctor about intimacy and sexual feelings?

In their book *Sexual Turning Points* (Macmillan, 1984), Lorna and Philip Sarrel explain that we tend to be afraid that others will be shocked or embarrassed if we bring up the subject of sex when we "should" be concentrating on our health and well-being—as though sex weren't a natural part of well-being. Some doctors may be uncomfortable with personal relationship questions. Fortunately, an increasing number of doctors will respond to direct questions about sexual function without embarrassment or shock. However, it's reasonable for you to say to your doctor: "I have concerns about the sexual part of my life. Is this a problem you can help me with or can you recommend someone for me to see?"

How do I find a professional sex therapist or counselor?

Usually, you can ask your physician or another health professional or minister to make a referral. The professionals most qualified to deal with your sexuality problems include psychiatrists (medical doctors who specialize in mental health), psychologists (people with a Ph.D. or M.A. in psychology), licensed marriage counselors, family therapists, and social workers. Those who are most highly trained usually belong to one or more of the following organizations: the American Association of Sex Educators, Counselors and Therapists, the American Association for Marriage and Family Therapy, the American Family Therapy Association, or the National Association of Social Workers. If your physician or other health professional or minister cannot make a referral, you can locate members of these organizations by looking in the Yellow Pages of your telephone directory under Marriage and Family Counseling, or by consulting the American Cancer Society or the Cancer Information Service.

What questions should I ask the therapist before starting treatment?

You can ask the therapist a number of questions to find out about professional training and counseling techniques. Some questions you might want answered include:

- What is your professional training and degree?
- Have you had training and experience in dealing with sexual problems relating to cancer?
- Do you usually see partners together or as individuals? (It is usually advisable in dealing with sexual problems for both partners to be together when advice is given.)
- How frequently will we meet?
- How long are the sessions?
- What does each session cost?
- Does insurance cover the cost?

What does a sex therapist do?

Sex therapists are trained to evaluate and treat sexual problems. Usually, a sex therapist wants to hear from both partners about problems and how each partner views them. Bringing problems into the open and discussing them with a professional can help put them into perspective so you can deal with them in a knowledgeable way.

Are there any suggestions for ways to make it easier to continue my sex life during or after cancer treatment?

Here are some thoughts that may be helpful:
- If you feel weak or tired and want your partner to take a more active role, or you just want to hug and caress, say so.
- Remember that no matter how ill you feel, the ability to feel pleasure from touching almost always remains.
- Time your sexual activity for the hours you feel best. If, for example, you are taking pain medication, take your medicine before you have sex. Be aware, however, that too much pain medication may decrease desire and interfere with the ability to achieve an erection or orgasm.
- Try to keep an open mind and be creative about ways to give and receive sexual pleasure. There may be times when intercourse is not possible, but you and your partner may still help each other feel satisfied through mutual caressing and stimulation.
- Try different positions and use pillows to make yourself more comfortable.
- Try different, less energetic types of sexual activity, such as massage, or self-stimulation.
- Taking a shower together can be physically relaxing and sexually stimulating.

How can a single person cope with the aloneness of cancer?

Being single and having cancer often makes you feel more alone than ever. So many loose ends in your life seem to be dangling. Your world seems to be filled with nothing but uncertainty. Your view of yourself may need to be repolished. You may feel that you have been robbed of your future. If you had hoped to marry or remarry, you may feel reluctant about starting a new relationship because you are not certain what the future will bring. Of course, there are no simple answers to how to go about regaining your verve for living and getting on with your life, but there's no better time than right now to work at developing a network of close, caring friends. Get involved in a hobby, special interest group, or a course of study that will help you to meet new people. Every town has many activities that are worthy of your interest. Check your newspapers for church groups, Y's, art centers, historical societies, or auto clubs for ideas of activities that might be of interest to you. Make a real effort to stay involved with friends, keeping in touch with telephone calls, planning visits and special events. And don't overlook support groups geared to people who have had cancer. If one does not already exist, you may want to consider starting your own self-help group for single people who have had cancer.

What and when do you tell someone new in your life about your cancer?

In dating relationships, most people who've had cancer frequently choose not to discuss their illness. The decision is often a difficult one, but many who have had cancer say that it is especially hard when you are trying to be at your very best in a new relationship to draw attention to your weaknesses. So the question becomes, when is the best time to tell? The answer that seems to work best for most people is that it is not necessary to discuss your cancer with every person you date, but when the relationship becomes serious, before you decide to make a strong commitment, it is wise to bring up the subject. Try to pick your moment at a time when you and your partner are relaxed. The words you use will be your own but it may be helpful to you to practice what you might say. Simple statements are best. "You know I had cancer several years ago. I really want to know if you have concerns about being committed to someone who has had this problem?"

Why do I feel that I'd rather not get involved with someone than be rejected?

This is not an uncommon feeling, but it is very counterproductive behavior. By not becoming involved, you are certain not to be rejected. But you are depriving yourself of all the good times you could be having. Think about it. It isn't only people with cancer who are rejected. It happens to everyone at some time in their lives. Romantic relationships between healthy people frequently break up. It's unfortunate to reject the opportunity to form new relationships on the outside chance you might be rejected. If this is difficult for you to resolve, a brief session or two with a therapist may help you to feel more comfortable with the changes in your body, and give you skills to cope more successfully with yourself.

Is there any way to remove a scar that makes me feel sexually unattractive?

Some scars can be camouflaged with makeup. There are several brands of heavier makeup specifically designed for this, such as Covermark, Dermablend, and Natural Cover, which are available in department stores, beauty-supply houses, or by mail order. This makeup is designed to sit on top of the skin rather than blend into it. Theatrical makeup is also a possibility. It is possible that once healed, the scar may be removed with cosmetic surgery or some other method such as collagen injection. Be sure to discuss the possibilities with your doctor, who can recommend a qualified plastic surgeon.

What special beauty information is available for cancer patients?

There is a nationwide public service program designed to help people recovering from cancer deal with the changes in their appearances that may result from chemotherapy or radiation treatments or from the illness itself, such as loss of hair, eyebrows and lashes, changes in skin tone and texture or brittleness of nails. The program was developed by the Cosmetic, Toiletry and Fragrance Association Foundation as a partnership of the cosmetics industry, the American Cancer Society, and the National Cosmetology Association. The American Cancer Society, along with cancer centers and hospitals, runs the program locally with members of the National Cosmetology Association, offering their services on a voluntary basis to help patients learn the makeup techniques. A videotape (featuring makeover demonstrations on recovering cancer patients), workbooks, and brochures show makeup and hairstyling techniques. The volunteers give person-to-person, practical advice about appearance changes, including specific recommendations for skin care, hair styles, wigs and accessories, eyebrow and eye makeup, and nail care. To get information, call the local office of the American Cancer Society or the Cosmetic, Toiletry and Fragrance Association at 1-800-558-5005, or write to the Foundation at 1110 Vermont Avenue, NW, Suite 800, Washington DC 20005.

Sexuality and Chemotherapy

Chemotherapy can have side effects which may affect your sexuality. The one most dreaded by both women and men is the loss of hair. You may also gain or lose weight. You may feel tired and lack energy. In addition, there are a number of subtle biological and psychological side effects that are sometimes difficult to understand, but that may affect your sexual life. Knowing what to expect can help. Sense of touch may be dulled to near numbness or sharpened to the point of pain, resulting in a slower response or a feeling that the intensity of the response is uncomfortable. Changes in liver function and the metabolism of sex hormones can also be responsible for changes in response. It is comforting to know that many of these changes are temporary and will disappear when your treatments are completed.

What can be done about hair loss?

First of all, find out from your doctor whether the type of chemotherapy you will be having causes hair loss. Many chemotherapy drugs do not. If your doctor feels that you will be needing a wig, you may want to be prepared by shopping for one before you need it so you can match your own hair as closely as possible. Some people find this a good time to let their fantasies of having a different hair color run wild and choose several different colors of wigs. Women with long hair sometimes have their hair cut and have wigs made from their own hair. You may find it more comfortable to use your wig for outside appearances and wear a scarf, turban, or hat in the privacy of your home.

Are sexual relations harmful when you're undergoing chemotherapy?

There is no reason for sexual relations to hurt you when you are receiving chemotherapy, though touch perception—the way touch feels—can change as a result of the changes in your body chemistry. Of course, a great deal depends on where the cancer is and what stage it is in.

Is it normal for my emotions to swing from depression to real highs because of chemotherapy?

Although such emotional highs and lows are not unusual, it is important to report them to your doctor. It is imperative to determine if the mood swings are the result of the medications or of the emotions you feel about having cancer. Undergoing chemotherapy causes unusual stress. Often these side effects subside and moodiness disappears. However, if the quality of your life is being seriously changed by medication-related depression, your doctor may wish to adjust your medication schedule.

Is the menstrual cycle usually affected by chemotherapy?

Some drugs may change the menstrual cycle. Periods may come earlier or later than is usual for you and may last longer than normal. Some women's periods stop temporarily or they may stop altogether and cause menopausal symptoms such as hot flashes.

What are the symptoms of premature menopause?

The shortage of hormones in your body causes your periods to cease and you may be bothered by frequent hot flashes, especially at night. Some women also feel irritable and less interested in sex. Replacement hormones in a pill, shot, or vaginal cream can help with vaginal dryness and hot flashes. If your cancer is sensitive to estrogens, as are some tumors of the breast, uterus, or other genital areas, your doctor will probably avoid prescribing replacement hormones, since the estrogens could make any remaining cancer cells grow. If your doctor feels hormones would not be advisable for you, hot flashes can also be treated with drugs that control the nervous system's reactions to lack of estrogen.

> *"I lost my interest in sex—had premature menopause. Even now, four years later, I don't get aroused. I'm planning to see our family therapist about this. I don't understand why I have no interest. I do want to be held and massaged but nothing more."*
>
> *Diagnosed with lymphoma in 1984 at age 38*

Is it all right for me to become pregnant while I'm on chemotherapy?

If you are of childbearing age, it is important to discuss the subject of birth control and childbearing with your doctor. You should not become pregnant while you are on chemotherapy. Prevention is crucial because even if your periods stop, it is possible for you to conceive. Chemotherapy drugs are very powerful and harmful to the fetus, so it is vital to prevent pregnancy during chemotherapy treatment. Once treatment is completed, your menstrual periods may return and you may be able to conceive and have a normal pregnancy.

Can chemotherapy drugs damage the ovaries?

Many chemotherapy drugs can either temporarily or permanently damage the ovaries, reducing their output of hormones and affecting fertility. However, pregnancy may still be possible even if the menstrual cycle is disrupted, so birth control should not be overlooked.

Is it common to have a vaginal infection due to chemotherapy?

Since chemotherapy can lower the body's ability to fight infection, some women have vaginal yeast or bacterial infections which produce intense itching or burning sensations on the vulva or just inside the vagina. In some cases, the male partner also reacts, developing itching, burning, or redness of the penis after intercourse. It's a good idea to have vaginal infection symptoms checked by your doctor so proper treatment can be prescribed. To lessen irritation and prevent infection, wear cotton underwear rather than that made of synthetic fabric, panty hose with a ventilated crotch, and avoid shorts or slacks that are restricting.

Is there a reason why I have black and blue bruises from chemotherapy?

Low blood platelet counts are a side effect of many chemotherapy drugs. Low platelet counts may cause bruises or may cause you to bruise more easily. Strenuous sexual activity, when you are so susceptible to bruising, can result in black and blue marks on sensitive parts of your body. Women should use a lubricant during intercourse to avoid injury to vaginal tissues while platelet counts are low.

Is vaginal dryness a side effect of chemotherapy treatments?

Cancer treatments often reduce the amount of moisture your vagina produces, so you may need extra lubrication to make intercourse comfortable. A water-based lubricant, such as KY Jelly, Lubrifax, or Ortho Personal lubricant, can help. Vaseline is not recommended because it is oil-based and can increase the chance of vaginal infection. Your physician may want to check your estrogen level to see whether the dryness is due to a physical change in your ovaries or vagina.

What effect does chemotherapy have on male sexual organs?

Often, men who are undergoing chemotherapy have a reduced sperm count, sometimes resulting in sterility. This, of course, does not mean that erection or intercourse is affected. Sperm production may return to normal when chemotherapy is completed, although in some cases men may be permanently sterile. It is advisable to use contraceptive precautions while you are on chemotherapy.

Can sperm be stored for future use?

For men desiring children, freezing or storing sperm for future use, prior to chemotherapy treatments, may be an option if there is a possibility of sterility from treatment. This alternative should be discussed with the medical staff before treatment. Unfortunately, the technique is not always successful since the quality of sperm may be such that conception may not occur. Production of sperm may return when chemotherapy treatments are stopped, although it is possible that sperm counts and the effectiveness of the sperm may be permanently reduced by some drugs.

How does chemotherapy affect male sexual desire?

Sexual desire often decreases immediately after a course of chemotherapy but usually recovers after a few weeks. Chemotherapy can occasionally affect sexual desire and erections by slowing down testosterone production. Medications used to prevent nausea can upset your hormonal balance, though hormone levels usually return to normal after treatments are over. There is some evidence that chemotherapy drugs such as cis-platinum or vincristine can permanently damage parts of the nervous system, and it is believed that these nerves may have some control over erections, though there is no scientific proof that this is the case.

How can you camouflage a permanent chemotherapy catheter implanted in the shoulder or arm?

High-necked tops or long sleeves can help hide the catheter but may be uncomfortable in warm weather. Cotton or silk fabrics are more porous than synthetics and will feel cooler.

Sexuality and Radiation

Lots of people who have cancer undergo radiation treatment. There are two kinds—external and internal—and to most people, radiation therapy seems like the easiest sort of treatment. It's fast and it's painless. The cumbersome machinery used can be intimidating. The whole business of marking the body with indelible ink makes people feel like they're being tattooed. But once they realize that the machinery is shielded and all the safeguards involved are for their own protection, most people manage to tolerate radiation without too many problems, although they may feel more tired than usual.

Many people worry that radiation treatments will leave them radioactive. The radioactivity of external radiation is confined to the treatment beam itself. Neither the normal tissues nor the cancerous ones become radioactive. When the treatment is completed, no radioactivity remains in the body.

Those who have internal radiation treatments—either where the radioactive material is sealed in a container and inserted in the body or where it is given orally or injected in a syringe to get the radioactive material as close to the tumor as possible—usually have some restrictions placed on them during the time they are being treated. The restrictions depend upon the kind of radioactive material, the location, and the dose. Generally, young visitors and those who are pregnant are not allowed in the room until the radioactive material has been removed or is no longer radioactive.

Will radiation cause physical changes that lead to sexual problems?

This will depend on exactly where you are being radiated. Radiation therapy to male or female sexual organs, for example, may cause some problems. External-beam radiation to the prostate area can cause impotence as well as decreased sexual desire—often temporarily. In women, radiation to the pelvic area can cause narrowing, dryness, and thinning of the vagina. Itching of the dry areas is also common. During radiation, tissues in the target area become irritated and inflamed, as they do with a serious sunburn. A woman's vagina may feel tender during radiation treatment and for a few weeks afterwards. As the irritation heals, scarring occurs. The thick walls of the vagina may become "fibrous" and tough and lose some of their elasticity. Some women notice some light bleeding after intercourse, or ulcers or sore spots may develop in the area. In men, radiation may affect erection by damaging the arteries that carry blood to the penis. As the irradiated zone heals, internal tissues become scarred. The walls of the arteries may lose their elasticity and may no longer expand enough to let blood flow in to produce a firm erection.

Can I become sterile from radiation treatment?

This will depend on the dose of radiation and the location of treatment. If your sexual organs are in or close to the field of radiation, the treatment may cause sterility. If sterility is expected to result, whether you are a man or a woman, you should discuss the consequences with your doctor. Men may want to explore the possibility of having semen frozen and stored at a sperm-banking facility so that they may possibly have children later on. In women patients, it is sometimes possible to block or move the ovaries before radiation to protect them from exposure.

Is it common to have urinary-tract infections from radiation?

About one third of women who receive radiation therapy develop radiation cystitis—bladder irritation due to radiation. This is because the tissues become very sensitive as a result of treatment. Intercourse may cause the tissue surrounding the urethra to become swollen, inflamed, and susceptible to infection. The condition usually disappears four to six months following treatment.

Will I make my partner radioactive if I have sex after radiation treatments?

If you are having external radiation therapy, you are not radioactive and will not be a danger to anyone around you. There is no reason not to have intercourse if it is comfortable for you. If you are having internal radiation therapy, precautions are taken until the implants are removed or are no longer emitting radioactivity. You will be in the hospital during that time and will be given careful instructions.

Do radium implants in the prostate cause any aftereffects?

Radioactive implants in the prostate, though they require major abdominal surgery, usually result in few aftereffects. Once healing is completed, the quality of male erection is generally unaffected by the procedure. As with other forms of radioactive implants, there should be no fears of radiation aftereffects since the life of the radiation implant diminishes quickly (usually before the patient leaves the hospital).

How does radiation therapy for cancer of the penis, testicle, or prostate affect sterility or sexual performance?

It is known that fertility is affected, since the body often stops producing sperm. Usually, sperm production will begin again within six months to several years after treatment, though radiation therapy close to sexual organs can sometimes cause permanent sterility. As insurance, it is advisable to discuss the possibility of sperm banking before your treatments if you are interested in having children. Your doctor can check sperm count to determine the quality of sperm and how much is being produced.

Is painful ejaculation caused by radiation?

After radiation to the prostate, some men ejaculate only a few drops of semen. Toward the end of radiation treatments, men often feel a sharp pain as they ejaculate. This pain results from irritation in the urethra; it should fade within several months after the end of treatment.

Sexuality and Breast Cancer

For women, any breast surgery—especially when the entire breast is removed—is probably the most dreaded type of cancer surgery because it takes away such an important and visible part of the body, so closely allied to all of the feelings about sex and sexuality. Emotional recovery after breast surgery is as important a part of the recovery period as is the healing of the wound. Often the emotional scars remain long after the wound has healed. Expressing your feelings, even your most negative feelings, is part of the healing process, and is necessary to making a successful adjustment.

Why do they insist you look at your breast surgery scar before leaving the hospital?

Looking at your scar is part of the healing process. Your doctor and nurses are attempting to help you accept your loss. Often this is done by showing you how to care for your incision, thus giving you your first look at your scar. This is a very hard time for all breast patients, but when the swelling goes down and the scar heals completely, you'll begin to feel better able to cope. Being able to talk about your feelings will help, too. Until you are able to accept yourself and the changes in your body, it may be difficult for you to resume sexual intimacy.

Is it legitimate for me to fear my partner's getting near me because of my dread that he will hurt my incision?

This is a natural fear. However, the body's ability to heal is quite rapid, and you should try to relax and allow yourself to try to start getting back to normal without putting up barriers to resuming sexual relations. Intimacy can help to make you feel better psychologically. Be honest, explain your fears, and enlist your partner's help.

Why is it that, since my mastectomy, I seem to be having difficulties with my partner—having sex less often and not enjoying it as much?

Numerous studies have shown that some, but certainly not all, women who have had a mastectomy face a variety of problems involving sexuality. Some of the reasons include:
- You may be afraid of having your partner see your scars.
- You may be embarrassed to have your partner see you with only one breast.

- You may feel you will never be the same person sexually as you were before.
- Since breasts and nipples are important sources of sexual pleasure for many women, you fear you can't enjoy sex as before.
- Your partner may be afraid of causing you pain.
- The emotional problems may be more involved and more long-standing than the removal of your breast.

For some women, the loss is so great and so overwhelming that they cannot overcome it alone. If you are having problems of this kind, it is important for you to get some counseling or professional help. Mutual help groups can be enormously helpful.

"Sexual problems included a temporary awkwardness in our love relationship. It was my own self-doubts about my image as a woman who had lost a breast and my husband's concerns about my feelings and his own that made it hard. An excellent psychotherapist helped me work through my problems of low self-esteem that resulted from my breast operation."

Breast cancer, 1971, at age 46

Why is it that I coped perfectly well in the hospital but fell apart when I was home a few weeks?

Physical recuperation from the operation is usually quicker than psychological recovery. Very often the waves of feeling don't overwhelm you until you are home, where you feel everything is the same but you are different. Be patient with yourself. Realize that this is a normal part of recovery. Your recovery and readjustment will take time. Discuss your feelings as fully as you can with your partner, family, and close friends, and enlist their help. Try to get back to your normal routine as soon as possible, but don't rush it. Remind yourself that the loss of your breast, while changing your body image, has not changed the basic YOU.

Is it a normal sensation to feel that my breast is still there?

The so-called phantom breast sensation is experienced by many women who have undergone mastectomy. This can also include the feeling of pain in the missing breast, numbness, or a pins and needles feeling. It may last from a few weeks to many years.

What kind of positive things can I do to reaffirm my perception of my body image?

Physical exercise, such as tennis, swimming, dancing classes, or exercise classes, can help to improve your feelings about yourself. Your sense of balance and grace can be enhanced through dance-exercise classes. Yoga has been recommended as a way of achieving a sense of wholeness about the body. Many women have taken up such challenging new activities as skiing or racquetball. Others have returned to college and found a whole new sense of self-worth. Creative activities such as music, painting, stitchery, needlepoint, and writing are excellent fields to explore to help to get you back into the swing of things. You may find that joining a support group where you can discuss your feelings with other women who have shared your experience can help.

Should I explore the possibility of having my breast reconstructed?

This is a very personal decision and depends upon many factors. Some women who have had breast reconstruction tell us it has had a very positive effect, changing how they feel about themselves and affecting the way they feel about their sexual life as well. Others we know have said they don't want to go through further surgery and feel perfectly comfortable with themselves and with their partners.

Though reconstructed breasts cannot exactly duplicate the original, surgeons are now able to reconstruct the breast, the nipple, and areola. Not having to be concerned with a prosthesis and the unbalanced feeling of having only one breast has made this a good decision for some women.

Why is it so difficult to start an intimate relationship with a new man after breast surgery?

Before you can expect someone else to become accustomed to the idea of your breast surgery, you must come to grips with your own feelings of self-rejection. These very normal feelings hamper your self-image and make it hard for you to move into new intimacies. Breast surgery can be so shattering that you may have the impression that you are simply masquerading as normal. You may find it necessary to risk rejection from a man as part of your emotional healing process. You will learn, through this risk, that you are still a desirable, attractive, sensual woman. Be sure that you are not giving the wrong signals to a new partner. We know one man who told us how relieved he was to learn of his girlfriend's breast cancer. He had feared that she was a lesbian because of her seeming lack of interest in him. Becoming comfortable with the changes in your body will make it easier for you to become physically open with a man. One of the exercises that may help you is to study yourself in the nude before a mirror. Take time to get used to the way your changed body looks. Most scars are quite smooth and neatlooking. Feeling comfortable with the changes, accepting them, will make it possible for you to allow a man to get close to you so that you may enjoy an intimate relationship.

Sexuality and Female Sexual Organs

Cancer operations in the vaginal area often are a mystery to the women who have them since many of us have only a vague idea of how each of these parts of the body relates to the rest. You will find it very helpful to try to familiarize yourself completely with what has been done to you in your operation, become accepting of the changes that have occurred, and keep an open mind about enjoying sexual pleasures.

How does a total hysterectomy affect my lovemaking abilities?

Some women relax more and enjoy better orgasms because they no longer are worried about becoming pregnant. They report that lovemaking becomes more spontaneous and pleasurable. Other women report vaginal dryness associated with hormonal changes. This can often be corrected either with a water-soluble lubricant, estrogen creams, or estrogen supplements. The loss of ovarian androgens, affecting the supply of testosterone (the sexuality hormone), and/or the loss of the cervix and uterus (important in the sexual response of some, but not all, women) can also cause changes in sexual response. Although for many women the clitoris is more vital to female orgasm than the cervix and uterus, it is known that for some women, the quality of the orgasm seems to be related to the movement of the cervix and uterus and may be altered when these are removed.

"My libido dropped to almost nothing during treatment and it didn't return for three years. I talked to a sex therapist and he explained that some treatments change your sexual drive. That helps me to cope—just knowing."

Ovarian cancer, stage II, 1979, at age 29

What happens to me sexually when the ovaries are removed?

As far as your ability to engage in sexual activity is concerned, there are no physical reasons why you cannot continue in your usual manner, though a decrease in vaginal lubrication may make it necessary to use extra lubrication during intercourse. Because the ovaries are not the only production site for estrogens—the adrenal glands also produce androgens which govern sexual desire—there should be no change in your desire. When the ovaries are removed or destroyed, either by surgery or radiation, menopause occurs, often bringing with it hot flashes or other symptoms which may be more severe than those that accompany naturally occurring menopause. For women of childbearing age, this can be an emotionally difficult time, for they must come to grips with the fact that they can no longer have children.

What treatment is there for vaginal stenosis?

Vaginal stenosis, narrowing of the muscles and tissues that form the walls of the vagina, sometimes results from treatment. The tissues of the vagina may develop scar tissue, narrowing the passage and preventing your partner from entering the vagina or making it difficult for you to have a vaginal exam. Vaginal stimulation can help to prevent this complication. Since intercourse and the physical movement associated with lovemaking will stretch the vaginal tissues and muscles and help prevent scar-tissue formation, it is beneficial to have intercourse as frequently as possible within six weeks of the time of your surgery. Some physicians prescribe a program of vaginal dilation using a vaginal dilator to stretch out the vagina. Using the dilator several times a week keeps your vagina from developing tight scar tissue as the area heals. If you go for several months without a sexual relationship, it becomes especially important to use the dilator to keep your vagina from closing.

What can be done about preventing vaginal pain during sexual activity?

Pain during intercourse is probably the most common sexual problem for women following gynecological surgery. Sexual activity may cause pain in the vagina itself or in the delicate tissues surrounding it. Some women's vaginas are shorter or narrower as a result of radiation. If enough natural lubrication is not produced to make the vagina slippery, intercourse can be dry and uncomfortable and leave a sensation of burning or soreness. The risk of repeated urinary-tract infections is also increased.

Spread a generous amount of water-based lubricating gel inside your vagina before having intercourse. Or try using Lubrin, a lubrication suppository that melts during foreplay. Make sure you are fully aroused before you have intercourse. It is only when you are highly excited that your vagina expands to its fullest length and width and the walls produce lubricating fluid. Let your partner know if any kind of touching causes pain and show him the positions that aren't painful. Try different positions, such as kneeling over your partner with your legs on either side of his body, or facing each other while lying on your side.

How can I teach myself to relax my vaginal muscles?

Once you've felt pain during intercourse, without realizing it, you may tighten the muscles that ring the entrance to the vagina each time you have intercourse, making it more painful. If you become aware of these muscles, you can learn to control them. They're the same muscles that control your flow of urine. Next time you urinate, try stopping the flow for a few seconds and notice how you do it. When you relax the muscles, the urine flows once again. You can practice the same tightening and relaxing of the muscles when you are not urinating once you understand how it feels. To exercise the muscle, tighten to the count of 3 and then relax. You should try to practice tightening and relaxing 10 times, once or twice a day.

During lovemaking, when you are both aroused, you have lubricated your vagina, and are ready for intercourse, take a few seconds to tense your vaginal muscles and then let them relax as much as possible before penetration. If you feel any pain, you can signal your partner so you can stop a moment to tighten up and then relax your vaginal muscles, proceeding gently and gradually.

Are there any medications that would be helpful in making me relax my vaginal area?

Medications, including antispasmodics and analgesics, are sometimes used to help relax the body before intercourse and prevent the tightening of pelvic muscles. You should consult your doctor or a sex therapist to determine if medication might be helpful for you.

Can reconstructive surgery be performed following vaginal surgery?

Just as women who have undergone mastectomies may have breast reconstruction, women who have vaginectomies or colpectomies may have plastic surgery to reconstruct the vagina. Women who have had vaginal reconstruction say that this follow-up surgery can be helpful in regaining former sensations and feelings. Reconstruction is often done in stages and may involve several separate surgeries done several weeks or months apart. Many physicians are recommending that plans be made for reconstruction prior to the original surgery, when possible.

Male Sexual Problems

Any surgery in the male sexual organs raises questions of the
ability to continue to have sexual relations. Sometimes sexual
functioning is affected on a temporary basis, other times on a
permanent basis. It is important for you to be straightforward
from the start, questioning your doctor about what is being
done to you, what techniques are to be used, what the alternatives are, what the possible side effects may be, and discussing what you learn and your feelings with your partner.
If you do not understand the medical terminology, don't be
afraid to ask for an explanation in "plain English." In this way
you will be able to avoid unexpected physical and psychological aftereffects. Even if you haven't done that from the very
beginning, there's no better time than right now to start.

If your sex life is not fulfilling because of your treatment,
you need to talk with your physician or a sex therapist about
what can be done to help you to share intimacy in the fullest
way possible. No matter what the results of your surgery, you
are no less passionate now than you were before and it is
always possible to have a mutually satisfying love relationship
if you are willing to have free, open, frank, and uninhibited
communication.

**Is it unusual to lose all interest in sex during or immediately
after having treatment for cancer in the male sexual
organs?**

It's difficult to maintain an interest in sex when you feel that
your life is threatened. Loss of desire can result from anxiety
and depression, from the stress of long-term treatment, from
nausea, and from pain. Furthermore, cancer treatments can
interfere with the normal hormonal balance, which can cause
a lessening of sexual desire. Fear of being unable to have an
erection is one of the most common problems.

Are orgasms usually affected by cancer surgery?

Orgasm, the sexual climax, when the nervous system causes intense pleasure to be registered in the genitals, can be felt even if nerve damage or blocked arteries prevent a man from getting erections. There's no question that the stress and physical pain involved with treatment can have an effect on sexual response. However, it's important to understand that the nerves that control sensation and muscle contractions of orgasm are rarely damaged by cancer treatment, unless major surgery has been done on sexual organs. Loss of genital sensation or the inability to reach climax are generally only seen in cases where a tumor has damaged the areas of the brain and spinal cord that control these sensations. Sometimes hormonal therapy for prostate cancer can affect orgasm. Some surgery leaves a male with a dry orgasm. However, even when sensitive areas of tissue in the genital area are removed, most men learn to experience orgasm again.

Why have I lost my ability to have an erection?

There are many reasons for a man to lose his ability to have an erection. It happens to most men at one time or another —even to those who don't have cancer. The emotional stress of having cancer, depression, being tired, trying too hard, worry, and alcohol, can all result in erection problems. Cancer surgery and treatments may interfere with erection by damaging pelvic nerves or pelvic blood vessels.

Will my sexual problems after cancer treatment be permanent?

Many of the sexual problems that men experience after cancer treatment are temporary. Pain that occurs with erec-

tion or ejaculation after pelvic surgery or radiation usually
lessens and disappears. However, some cancer treatments do
permanently alter sexual functioning. Often it varies from
one person to the next. Some recover erections after radical
prostatectomy, for example, others do not. Sometimes it
takes years before healing is complete. One way of judging
whether the change is permanent or temporary is to test if
your reactions vary depending upon circumstances. Do you
have trouble getting or keeping an erection every time you
have sex? Are you able to do better when you stimulate
yourself? Yes answers indicate that the problem may be temporary. If your sleep erections are firm and long-lasting, you
will know that physically you function well, and the problem
probably lies with stress or psychological pressures.

If after several months your problems persist, you should
speak to your doctor about special medical tests to determine
the cause. Sleep laboratories are sometimes used to check
your sleep erections. Doctors use various devices to determine whether there are sleep erections. Blood tests and X-
rays may also be used to test reflexes in the genital area.

**Is sexual counseling helpful even if I know I cannot experi-
ence normal sex?**

When a medical condition limits sexual function, sex therapy
can be helpful in teaching you and your partner to learn how
to enjoy sexual caressing without erections.

What changes occur sexually when semen is not ejaculated?

Some cancer surgery results in a loss of the ability to produce
semen. The sperm cells made in the testicles ripen, but then
they are reabsorbed into the body. In other operations, the
ability to ejaculate through the penis is lost. Ejaculation
occurs but it is directed backward into the bladder, rather
than forward through the urethra. This is known as retro-

grade ejaculation. The semen remains in the bladder until urination, and is carried out via that route, and the urine looks cloudy because semen is mixed with it. The man who ejaculates in this manner has the very same sensations during sex that he had before except that there is no discharge through the penis. Sperm cells can be recovered from a man's urine and used to inseminate a woman.

Do men who have testicular cancer lose their sexual ability?

When retroperitoneal lymph node dissection, the removal of lymph nodes in the abdomen, is performed on men with testicular cancer, often the nerves that control emission are damaged, causing retrograde ejaculation. Sometimes these nerves recover over a one- to three-year period and the ejaculation of semen resumes. Erections and ability to reach orgasm usually are not affected, although the intensity may be less.

If I ejaculate less fluid when I have an erection, does that mean I will be unable to father children?

Cancer treatment can interfere with ejaculation by damaging the nerves that control the prostate, seminal vesicles, and opening to the bladder, or by stopping production of semen in the prostate and seminal vesicles, thus limiting the amount of semen. As long as sperm is intact, the amount of fluid is not the determining factor. The sperm count makes a difference, but even the production of less sperm does not mean that you will be unable to father children. As far as your sexual enjoyment is concerned, the amount of fluid ejaculated should not cause noticeable changes for you or your partner.

What types of cancer surgery can interfere with erections?

There are various operations and treatments that can result in loss of sexual power. The removal of the prostate and seminal vesicles for prostate cancer; the removal of the bladder, prostate, upper urethra, and seminal vesicles for bladder cancer, which requires a urinary ostomy; the removal of the lower colon and rectum for colon cancer, requiring a colostomy; and the total pelvic exenteration, when both a urinary ostomy and a colostomy are required—all can interfere, at least temporarily, with sexual functioning. All of these operations can damage the nerves that control blood flow to the penis, which means that the message to start an erection is either weakened or may be lost. Usually a man has partial erections after such surgery. Some men recover full erections—but it may take six months to a year or more before the blood vessels are healed sufficiently to restore blood flow to the penis.

Does radiation therapy cause erection problems?

Radiation can affect erection by damaging the arteries that carry blood to the penis. As the area heals, internal tissues may become scarred, and the walls of the arteries may lose some elasticity, causing the erection to be less firm. Radiation may also hasten hardening of the arteries, which may narrow the pelvic arteries. Two thirds of those having radiation therapy find that there is no change in their ability to have erections. The remainder sometimes find that the change may develop gradually over the year or two following radiation. Those who have high blood pressure or who have been heavy smokers, because of the prior damage to the arteries, may be at higher risk for erection problems.

Does radiation cause pain or a lessening of the amount of semen produced?

Some men say that toward the end of radiation treatments, they feel a sharp pain as they ejaculate. The pain results from irritation in the urinary tube through the penis, and should fade gradually in the months following treatment. After radiation to the prostate, some men ejaculate only a few drops of semen.

What are the effects of chemotherapy on the ability to have children?

Often, men who are undergoing chemotherapy have a reduced sperm count, sometimes resulting in sterility. This, of course, does not mean that erection or intercourse is affected. Production of sperm may return to normal when chemotherapy is completed, though in some cases men have become permanently sterile. Since the effect of chemotherapy on the sperm and unborn child is not really fully known, contraceptive precautions should be taken during treatment.

Does chemotherapy cause erection problems?

Most men who have chemotherapy continue to have normal erections. However, chemotherapy can sometimes affect sexual desire and erections by slowing down testosterone production, and some of the medications used to prevent nausea can upset the hormonal balance.

Can hormone treatment have an effect on the ability to achieve an erection?

Hormone therapy is sometimes used in treating prostate cancer that has spread beyond the prostate gland, in an attempt to starve the cancer cells of testosterone. Sometimes an operation to remove both testicles is done to achieve the same effect. Other times a combination of the two treatments is used. The most common side effect from these treatments is a decrease in the desire for sex. Some men say that their desire is still strong, but they have a problem achieving erection. Other men are able to continue to have normal sexual relations despite the fact that their bodies are no longer manufacturing testosterone.

What are the chances of being able to have an erection after having treatment for prostate cancer?

The answer depends on the stage of your cancer and the type of treatment. It is an important question to discuss with your doctor. Some treatments such as radium implants and radiation are less drastic than surgery. These treatments are used in some early stages of prostate cancer. New surgical techniques are making it possible to preserve the ability to have an erection.

What are the aftereffects of total prostatectomy?

Although the cancer may be controlled, there are a number of important possible side effects:
• Since the prostate gland produces most of the fluid released at the time of sexual intercourse and climax, most patients are sterile following this operation, just as they would be following a vasectomy.

- Many of the nerves that are involved with sexual functioning may be damaged, so that following surgery, many patients are no longer able to have an erection. New surgery avoiding the pelvic plexus is being done by selected doctors to overcome this problem.
- Some patients find that the operation causes them to lose their ability to control urine. Strengthening of muscles through simple exercise during recovery can sometimes help to return control. Urinary sphincter implants are possible to help control incontinence.

Can a total prostatectomy be done without impairing the ability to have an erection?

Dr. Patrick C. Walsh, a surgeon at Johns Hopkins University Hospital in Baltimore, Maryland, has developed a way of removing the prostate which preserves potency by bypassing the intricate nerve branches of the pelvic plexus. This technique is now being adopted by many surgeons for patients with early-stage prostate cancer. Until the advent of this type of surgery, 90 percent of those having prostatectomies lost their sexual ability and 2 to 5 percent became incontinent as well.

Why are my erections weaker following cancer treatment?

Mild decreases in the intensity of erection seem to be more common in men whose cancer treatments interfere with ejaculation of semen. However, this condition is also noted by men as they age.

Is a feeling of pain at erection a normal side effect?

Irritation of the prostate gland or urethra from cancer treatment can cause painful ejaculation. Pain in the penis as it becomes erect is sometimes seen in men over 40 because of dense fibrous tissue that causes a curve or knot to develop. However, this condition, known as Peyronie's disease, does not appear to be related to the fact that you have cancer. But any sign of pain should be brought to the attention of your doctor.

Does removal of one testicle affect potency or fertility?

No. Providing the remaining testicle is normal, there should be no change in function. A gel-filled implant, which has the weight, shape, and texture of a normal testicle, can be inserted surgically, either at the time of the operation or later, to restore normal appearance. Since cancer of the testicle rarely involves more than one testicle, erection is usually still possible, although there may be a decrease in ejaculation.

What sexual problems result from surgery on the penis?

It depends on the extent of the surgery. If only part of the penis has been removed, you may still be able to achieve erection and have the ability to perform penile/vaginal intercourse to the point of ejaculation. You may also be able to achieve orgasm and ejaculation by stimulation of the remaining part of your penis.

How can I have an active sex life if I am unable to have intercourse?

Many men find that open communication between both partners is the key to finding the best techniques. What pleases each of you the most? What parts of your bodies are the most sensual? What really turns each of you on? Even if you are unable to achieve erection and orgasm, you may still derive great pleasure and satisfaction in satisfying your mate. Helping your mate to learn how to caress and manipulate you to maximum satisfaction will afford you great pleasure. Seeking to give each other the greatest sexual satisfaction you are capable of achieving is what love is all about. Your sex life may not be the same as before, but there are still ways for you to have an active sex life and sexual enjoyment. You can learn to use your hands and your mouth to stimulate your partner. You may still be able to ejaculate with a non-erect penis or may learn to experience orgasms in other ways. Additionally, there are several prosthetic devices which can be inserted surgically in the penis to make intercourse possible.

Are penile implants a satisfactory solution?

Many doctors are doing surgery to implant a prosthesis in the penis, called a penile implant. Several types of prostheses are available. Some are semi-rigid, others are inflatable. They are implanted inside the corpora cavernosa, two structures within the penis resembling long balloons that normally fill with blood during an erection. There are advantages and disadvantages to both the inflatable and semi-rigid types. The inflatable prosthesis gives a natural-looking appearance. The pump system is installed entirely within the body, and allows you to transfer fluid from a reservoir to two inflatable balloons that go into the penis. There are tubings from the pump to the reservoir. When deflation is desired, a valve on the side of the pump is pressed to release the fluid back into the reservoir. This type of prosthesis requires an extensive operation and, because it is mechanically complicated, there are potentials for problems once it is inserted. Corrections of problems may require further surgical procedures.

Another type of prosthesis is a semi-rigid device. Although it is easier to insert and hardly ever malfunctions, it is less satisfactory because once it is inserted, the penis remains in an erect position, and must be bent up or down to conceal it during daily activities.

Other Sexual Problems Caused by Specific Cancers

There are a number of types of cancer, other than those that are directly related to sexual organs, which may cause sexual problems. The way in which we will be accepted by our friends, lovers, family, and fellow workers following an operation that changes the way we look to others or the way we feel about ourselves reflects upon our sexual lives. Feelings about sexuality influence all the other parts of our lives, and so it is important to look at some of the other cancers that most obviously involve the way we feel about ourselves—facial cancers, cancers that involve the voice, limb amputation, and ostomy (an operation in which an artificial opening is made in the abdomen).

Before going any further to look at some of the specific problems, let's talk about the most basic factor in sexual intimacy: liking yourself. That feeling becomes contagious. If you feel good about yourself, others feel good about you. If you accept your changes, others will, too. As you become happier with yourself, you'll feel better about yourself and you'll find it easier to deal with problems and communicate your feelings to others.

"Amazingly enough, cancer changed my life. I know that each day is precious. We have resolved a bad marriage. We have worked through our problems and are able to love each other and show it again. I know what counts now. It isn't hair or money. It is loving and being loved."

Diagnosed with lymphoma in 1984 at age 38

Is it common to be depressed and unable to be involved in a sexual relationship when you've had surgery for facial cancer?

Many patients whose operation has caused facial disfigurement naturally go through some depressed periods. Because the scars are so public, there is no way of hiding them. However, recent advances in facial prostheses and in plastic surgery now give many people a more normal appearance and most are able to live their lives much as they did before. Special support and understanding from mates, family, and friends is needed during the difficult period of treatment and adjustment.

Do people who've had a laryngectomy have any special advice for making sexual encounters more pleasant?

Surgery that removes the voice box (laryngectomy) leaves you without the normal means of speech. Breathing is through an opening in the neck that is usually covered by a covering to catch dust and particles as well as mucus. During sexual activity, most people wear a cover. Care should be taken to minimize odors from the stoma by avoiding spicy or garlicky foods. Difficulty in speaking may interfere with communication during sex, but most people report that they learn to communicate with touch and that talking is not absolutely necessary in most sexual situations. Excellent information about all aspects of life as a laryngectomee is available through the International Association of Laryngectomees (IAL), which can be reached through your local American Cancer Society.

What kinds of sexual adjustments must you make when you've had a limb amputated?

The question of whether or not to wear the limb prosthesis during sex is much debated. Sometimes wearing the prosthesis helps with positioning and ease of movement, but the straps that attach it to the body can get in the way. Without the prosthesis, you may have trouble feeling balanced during intercourse. Pillows can be helpful when properly placed. Amputations may cause chronic pain or result in phantom limb sensations; these can interfere with sexual desire and distract you during lovemaking. Phantom pain usually disappears but it is important to deal with problems as they occur to keep pain patterns from becoming firmly established. Most people with limb amputations continue with their normal lives, overcoming the obstacles with courage and ingenuity.

Does having an ostomy mean giving up a sexual life?

Having an ostomy usually does not lessen a man's or a woman's capability to enjoy sex, though there may be psychological barriers that may make sexual adjustment difficult. You should be certain that the appliance fits properly. Avoid foods that are spicy or garlicky. Women may feel more comfortable wearing a filmy nightgown and men may prefer to cover the stoma with a T-shirt or undershirt. To minimize rubbing against the ostomy, choose positions for sexual activity that keep your partner's weight off it. A small pillow can be helpful to keep from rubbing the ostomy. Some men and women feel sexual pleasure when their ostomy is touched, and this is neither abnormal nor strange. But care must to taken in handling the stoma, since it is a delicate area and can become irritated if rubbed too strenuously. A great deal of excellent information about adjusting to an ostomy is available through the United Ostomy Association, 36 Executive Park, Suite 120, Irvine, CA 92714, 714-660-8624.

Checklist for Putting Your Relationship into Perspective

This is not a test. There is no passing or failing score. The statements merely highlight what is happening in your sexual life. If each partner checks off his/her answers separately, you can compare notes and use what you learn about each other to gain greater understanding. Two checklists are included—one for each partner. Check True, False, Don't Want to Discuss, or Doesn't Apply, for each statement.

QUESTIONNAIRE FOR YOURSELF

True	False	Don't Want to Discuss	Doesn't Apply	
				I want so much to share intimacy, but I'm not up to sexual intercourse.
				She/he doesn't seem interested in sex.
				I just don't seem to get sexually aroused.
				I'm afraid my partner will hurt me.
				I'm not interested anymore.
				I purposely avoid sex.
				Sex is unsatisfying for me.
				I'm satisfied with just being held and cuddled.
				I feel failure and inadequacy about sex.
				I wish we could be more frank and open.

TRUE	FALSE	DON'T WANT TO DISCUSS	DOESN'T APPLY	
				I get excited but don't reach a climax.
				Sex isn't what it used to be.
				I'm getting too old to enjoy sex.
				I can't seem to get an erection/climax so I avoid sex.
				I'm worried because my partner doesn't enjoy sex.
				My partner won't try anything different.
				I can't seem to get aroused no matter how hard I try.
				True love lasts a lifetime no matter what happens.
				I can't come to orgasm/climax when I want to.
				My illness has changed the way I see myself as a person.
				I'm not sure whether he/she is avoiding me, doesn't feel up to it, or just isn't interested anymore.
				Our loving has gotten very routine.
				I love sex and want to make it even better.
				I really used to enjoy sex but not anymore.
				Being ill has interfered with my being a husband/wife.
				Being ill has interfered with my being a mother/father.

True	False	Don't Want to Discuss	Doesn't Apply	
				I think it's time we faced the fact that we cannot have intercourse and discussed other means of physical interaction.
				I would be happy if he/she would talk with me honestly about how he/she feels about making love.
				I wish we could talk about the scariness of the diagnosis.
				He/she is sexually cold.
				He/she is uninterested.
				My partner is afraid of catching cancer.
				I'm convinced that radiation is harmful to me.
				I'm repelled by the operation and the changes in my body.
				I think my partner is selfish wanting sex when I am so ill.
				I think it's inappropriate to be thinking about sex in the midst of a life-threatening illness.
				He/she is indifferent.
				At this point, I'm willing to look upon our relationship as friendship/companionship and disregard the sexual factor.
				I'm willing to forgo the sexual factor in our relationship but I'd like to talk about it.

True	False	Don't Want to Discuss	Doesn't Apply	
				I find self-stimulation is a good sexual outlet for me.
				I've never tried masturbation.
				I think masturbation is abnormal.
				I'd be willing to try masturbation as an alternative.
				I'd like to try a vibrator.
				Change rarely occurs in a good relationship.
				Sickness changes things and makes ordinary things hard to deal with.
				Humor doesn't help when serious problems arise.
				Sex is still good, even though we have problems.
				We are better able to communicate with sex than with words.
				I'd be willing to try some different ways of making love.
				Our love doesn't have much meaning.
				Our love has changed.
				Our love has developed into deeper love.

After you have discussed your checklists together, you may want to try answering and talking about the following questions:

List three fears you had when you discovered you/your partner had cancer:

		Has the Fear	
		Increased?	Decreased?
1.	_____	_____	_____
2.	_____	_____	_____
3.	_____	_____	_____

On a scale of 1 to 10:

_____ • How satisfied are you with the quality of closeness you share?

_____ • How important is sexual intercourse to you as an expression of intimacy?

_____ • How important are other means of physical interaction to you?

What makes you feel most loved and appreciated? _____
_____

What was one recent circumstance that made you feel close to your partner? _____
_____
_____

What keeps you from becoming closer to your partner? _____
_____

What can your partner do to make you happier? _____
_____

What does your partner think are the things that make you happiest in your physical relationship? _____
_____

YOUR PARTNER'S QUESTIONNAIRE

True	False	Don't Want to Discuss	Doesn't Apply	
				I want so much to share intimacy, but I feel my partner is not up to sexual intercourse.
				She/he doesn't seem interested in sex.
				My partner just doesn't seem to get sexually aroused.
				I'm afraid of hurting him/her.
				I'm not interested anymore.
				I purposely avoid sex.
				Sex is unsatisfying for me.
				I'm satisfied with just being held and cuddled.
				I feel failure and inadequacy about sex.
				I wish we could be more frank and open.
				I get excited but don't reach a climax.
				Sex isn't what it used to be.
				I'm getting too old to enjoy sex.
				I can't seem to get an erection/climax so I avoid sex.
				I'm worried because my partner doesn't enjoy sex.
				My partner won't try anything different.

True	False	Don't Want to Discuss	Doesn't Apply	
				I can't seem to get aroused no matter how hard I try.
				True love lasts a lifetime no matter what happens.
				I can't come to orgasm/climax when I want to.
				The illness has changed the way my partner sees him- or herself as a person.
				I'm not sure whether he/she is avoiding me, doesn't feel up to it, or just isn't interested anymore.
				Our loving has gotten very routine.
				I love sex and want to make it even better.
				I really used to enjoy sex but not anymore.
				Being ill has interfered with my partner's being a husband/wife.
				Being ill has interfered with my partner's being a mother/father.
				I think it's time we faced the fact that we cannot have intercourse and discussed other means of physical interaction.
				I would be happy if he/she would talk with me honestly about how he/she feels about making love.
				I wish we could talk about the scariness of the diagnosis.
				He/she is sexually cold.

True	False	Don't Want to Discuss	Doesn't Apply	
				He/she is uninterested.
				I'm afraid of catching cancer.
				I'm convinced that my partner's radiation is harmful to me.
				I'm repelled by the operation and the changes in my partner's body.
				I don't want to seem selfish wanting sex when my partner is so ill.
				I think it's inappropriate to be thinking about sex in the midst of a life-threatening illness.
				He/she is indifferent.
				At this point, I'm willing to look upon our relationship as friendship/companionship and disregard the sexual factor.
				I'm willing to forgo the sexual factor in our relationship but I'd like to talk about it.
				I find self-stimulation is a good sexual outlet for me.
				I've never tried masturbation.
				I think masturbation is abnormal.
				I'd be willing to try masturbation as an alternative.
				I'd like to try a vibrator.
				Change rarely occurs in a good relationship.

True	False	Don't Want to Discuss	Doesn't Apply	
				Sickness changes things and makes ordinary things hard to deal with.
				Humor doesn't help when serious problems arise.
				Sex is still good, even though we have problems.
				We are better able to communicate with sex than with words.
				I'd be willing to try some different ways of making love.
				Our love doesn't have much meaning.
				Our love has changed.
				Our love has developed into deeper love.

After you have discussed your checklists together, you may want to try answering and talking about the following questions:

List three fears you had when you discovered you/your partner had cancer:

	Has the Fear Increased?	Decreased?
1. _____	_____	_____
2. _____	_____	_____
3. _____	_____	_____

On a scale of 1 to 10:

_____ • How satisfied are you with the quality of closeness you share?

_____ • How important is sexual intercourse to you as an expression of intimacy?

_____ • How important are other means of physical interaction to you?

What makes you feel most loved and appreciated? _____

_____

What was one recent circumstance that made you feel close to your partner? _____

_____

_____

What keeps you from becoming closer to your partner? _____

_____

What can your partner do to make you happier? _____

_____

What does your partner think are the things that make you happiest in your physical relationship? _____

_____

Things to Say to Your Partner Who Has Cancer

- We're in this together.
- I'm here to do anything and everything I can to help you.
- Lean on me. I'll be here to give you strength.
- I married you for better and for worse, in sickness and in health, till death do us part.
- I love you—and I'll be with you all the way.
- Don't panic. Let's just take it step by step and day by day.

chapter 5

Learning More About Diet and Nutrition

Every magazine you pick up seems to have another article on proper diet and nutrition. Health food stores abound. Books on the subject fill the bookshelves. Studies are being conducted at many different levels to determine the effect of various foods and vitamins. The desire for health and fitness, the uncertainty about the safety of many foods, the seductiveness of diets that are presented to us as cure-alls, can all combine to leave us in a muddle about what we should be eating. People who are in the process of being treated for cancer need a well-balanced diet to help maintain strength so that the body will be able to help in the fight to rid itself of cancer cells.

It's important to look at scientific evidence in gauging the value of diets, supplements, and other advice concerning nutrition. Don't be led down the garden path of promise by relying on therapies that are supposed to "cleanse the body of poisons," but merely end up washing out essential nutrients. Be careful about taking vitamins and minerals that may distort the body's nutritional balance or cause druglike side effects. Look long and carefully at any supposed cure that is based on a specific diet. There is a great deal of well-documented evidence that you would be wise to study in making your decisions about your diet. Self-education is important. Be warned, however, that findings are often contradictory or inconclusive. Some principles and theories are better reasoned than others. Because the issue is so complex and important, only a qualified dietician, nutritionist, or nutrition-oriented physician can intelligently advise you about making any major changes in your diet.

Can I go to my doctor for information about what diet is best for me?

Although you will want to let your oncologist know your concerns about improving your diet, don't be surprised if your request is met in a noncommittal, half-hearted, or even hostile way. Many traditional doctors still are not educated in nutrition and some can be quite antagonistic about the whole subject. More and more doctors, however, realizing the heightened public interest in nutrition as it relates to health, are advising their patients to seek nutritional help.

How do I go about finding a good nutritionist?

Many people call themselves nutritionists who are not. Nutritionists need a background in biochemistry to understand the subtleties of nutrition and make intelligent decisions about a person's needs. Since only 13 states license or certify nutritionists, finding a good nutritionist on your own can be a problem. Most of the legitimate ones are registered dieticians (RDs), which means they have been certified by the American Dietetic Association. To be certified, they must be college graduates, complete an internship in nutrition counseling or food service management, pass a national exam, and take 75 hours of courses every five years. There are about 47,000 registered dieticians in the United States, some of whom are employed by hospitals, clinics, and beauty spas. There are also M.D.s with postgraduate training and clinicians with Ph.D.s in nutrition. They are usually members of the American Society of Clinical Nutrition and certified by the American Board of Nutrition. A lack of registered credentials doesn't necessarily mean a lack of competence, but it does mean you should check out reputation by other means.

Here are some ways of searching out nutritionists in your area:

- Ask a doctor, nurse, or local hospital for a recommendation. Many food counselors work in conjunction with the medical profession, providing special help for patients.
- Look in the Yellow Pages of your telephone directory under Nutrition. Listed there you will probably find a number of names, only a few of whom will be Ph.D.s or registered dieticians. Some counselors will have M.S. after their names, indicating an advanced degree in science. Nutrition counselors and clinical nutritionists are common listings, but this does not give you much information as to qualifications except by omission.
- Questionable credentials include a degree in nutrition counseling from unaccredited correspondence schools or degree initials such as N.D., Doctor of Naturopathy; C.H., Certified Herbologist; or R.H., Registered Healthologist. Listings offering nutritional and metabolic evaluation services such as hair analyses and cytotoxic blood tests for determining food sensitivities are widely questioned.
- You can learn a great deal by making telephone calls and speaking with counselors, asking questions about qualifications and background, how long they have been counseling, what types of patients they usually work with, what kind of treatment and testing, if any, is used. These will give you some subtle clues as to legitimacy. Be sure to ask what the charges will be and how many visits most patients average. Services may vary from $30 to $100 per hour. Usually two visits are sufficient for nutrition counseling. Few people need more than six sessions unless there are complex problems.
- Be wary of counselors who suggest megadoses of vitamins and minerals or who sell the remedies prescribed. Most

reputable nutritionists prescribe vitamins and minerals sparingly, concentrating on sharpening your nutritional skills instead.

Are there special nutrition requirements for people undergoing treatment?

Good nourishment is needed for healing and building new tissues. People who eat well during treatment, especially foods high in protein and calories, are better able to stand the side effects of treatment. Some researchers feel it may even be possible for these patients to withstand a higher dose of certain treatments. There are nutrition experts who believe that during chemotherapy, for example, you may need as much as 50 percent more protein than usual and 20 percent more calories. People with good eating habits tend to have fewer infections and are often able to be up and about more. When a person eats less, for whatever reason, the body uses its own stored-up fat, protein, and other nutrients, such as iron. However, it is often difficult, if not impossible, to fulfill the requirements of a so-called balanced diet even when your health is good and your appetite is at its peak. Many people having chemotherapy or radiation therapy lose interest in food during treatment, which creates additional problems. If your appetite is poor when you are undergoing treatment, you need to make sure that the food you are eating is high in protein and calories and that you are attentive to the need for eating well.

What is meant by eating well when you are undergoing treatment?

You need to try to have a diet that is high enough in calories to keep up your normal weight, if at all possible. Eat any time you're hungry. Try to eat the most nutritious, caloric foods. People who have had surgery or are undergoing treatment need extra protein and other nutrients for repairing their body tissues. Try to eat foods that are high in protein, since protein can be used for repair if the body is also getting enough calories. If it is not, the body will use the protein for energy instead of repair. Try to eat a varied diet. The National Cancer Institute has a number of fine publications which can be helpful during treatment. *Chemotherapy and You* and *Radiation Therapy and You*, as well as *Eating Hints*, are all available to you by calling the Cancer Information Service at 1-800-4-CANCER.

"I feel nutrition is very important and made a promise to myself to maintain the best nutrition possible. I was already on a diet for duodenal ulcers so I make myself eat correctly."

Modified radical mastectomy, 1987, at age 67

Are there guidelines on how much protein and how many calories are required during recuperation?

During illness, treatment, and recovery, it is estimated that women need about 80 grams of protein (compared to a normal daily need of 44 grams) and men require 90 grams (compared to a normal daily need of 46 grams). An additional 200 to 300 calories should also be added to the diet. If your weight is stable, chances are that you do not need to increase your intake. If you are losing weight, you should add protein and calories to your diet.

How can I add protein to my diet?

You can add protein to the diet in several ways without increasing the amount of food you eat. For example:
- Add skim milk powder to the regular milk you use in recipes. Two tablespoons can give you added protein.

- Fortify the milk you drink by adding one cup of instant non-fat dry milk to every quart of milk (homogenized or low fat). Beat the milk after adding the dry milk to make sure it is dissolved. Chill for several hours to improve flavor.
- Add milk powder to hot or cold cereals, scrambled eggs, soups, gravies, casserole dishes, and desserts.
- Add diced or ground meat to soups and casseroles.
- Add grated cheese or chunks of cheese to sauces, vegetables, soups, and casseroles.
- Add cream cheese or peanut butter as well as butter to your bread.
- Choose dessert recipes that contain eggs—such as sponge and angel food cake, egg custard, bread pudding, or rice pudding.
- Add peanut butter to sauces. Use it on crackers, waffles, or celery sticks.

How can I add calories to my diet?

Again, there are ways to increase calories without increasing the amount of food you eat:
- Mix butter into hot foods such as soups, vegetables, mashed potatoes, cooked cereal, and rice. A teaspoon of butter or margarine will add 45 calories.
- Use mayonnaise instead of salad dressing in salads or on sandwiches. Mayonnaise adds 100 calories per tablespoon.
- Use peanut butter on fruits, such as apples, bananas, or pears. Layer celery with peanut butter for a snack. Add it to a sandwich with cream cheese. One tablespoon of peanut butter has 90 calories and is also rich in protein.
- Try sour cream or yogurt on vegetables such as potatoes, beans, carrots, or squash. Use them on gravies or as a salad dressing for fruit. One tablespoon of sour cream has 70 calories.
- Add whipping cream to pies, fruit, puddings, hot chocolate, Jello, or other desserts. One tablespoon adds 60 calories.

- Prepare snacks and have them ready to eat. Nuts, dried fruits, candy, popcorn, crackers and cheese, granola, ice cream, and popsicles all make good snacks. Milk shakes add calories and are easy to make with a blender.
- Add raisins, dates, or chopped nuts and brown sugar to hot cereals or to cold cereals for a snack.

Should I be worried about the amount of fat in my diet while I am undergoing treatment?

That is a difficult question to answer. Fats are the most concentrated source of energy. They give about twice the number of calories as do an equal weight of protein or carbohydrates. Therefore, nutritionists believe that if you need additional calories, the most efficient way to get them is by adding fat to the diet. If your body is not getting enough calories, it will use protein for energy instead of using it for repairing body tissues. So it is important to be sure you are getting enough calories during the time you are undergoing treatment, be it surgery, chemotherapy, radiation therapy or immunotherapy.

Doesn't fat cause cancer?

There is some research which shows that eating too much fat may increase your chance of getting cancers of the colon, breast, prostate, and endometrium. However, you need to look at the requirements your body has while you are undergoing treatment versus the diet you might want to follow for the rest of your life. You need to weigh the importance of making sure your body is well nourished to help you get through the treatments and help you decrease the severity and duration of side effects as opposed to what you will do in the long term after your treatment has finished.

Should I also be taking extra vitamins and minerals?

Some researchers suggest adding vitamins and minerals to the nutritional regimen to help protect the body, during and following surgery, from the toxicity of drugs and to help improve the functioning of the immune system. It's important to distinguish between reasonably large doses of vitamins and vitamin megadosing. You might ask your doctor or nutritionist about taking injectable vitamins as a way of boosting vitamin efficiency.

Does anyone really know what vitamins and minerals and in what amounts are best for you?

What to take and how much to take have always been the subject of controversy. People recovering from injuries or surgery have greatly increased requirements for certain vitamins. People who smoke, drink moderate amounts of alcohol, or take oral contraceptives also need more vitamins than they otherwise would and may undergo vitamin depletion even when their vitamin intake is adequate for normal people. The B-complex vitamins are essential in the process by which food is used for energy, repair, and all the other essentials of life. Vitamin C is necessary, among other things, for the body to make collagen, a major component of skin, tendons, and bones. The body depends on vitamin A for healthy epithelial tissue—that is, the tissue that forms the covering or lining of all body surfaces, including the lining of the digestive tract, the lungs, the blood vessels, and so on. Vitamin E is an antioxidant; it protects lipids (water-soluble fats) from the attack of oxidizing agents of all sorts. Potassium deficiencies can result from diarrhea or vomiting. Attention should be paid to increasing potassium either through supplements or by adding potassium-rich foods like potatoes, molasses, raisins, or bananas to the daily diet.

Is there a difference in nutritional needs once treatment is completed?

During treatment, your body needs extra protein and calories to help in the healing process. Once that's all behind you, you'll want to learn about diet and nutrition as it relates to cancer prevention. (This is discussed later in the chapter.) Although there is little research on whether or not nutrition can prevent recurrence, more and more evidence is being gathered through animal studies and studies of large population groups that correlates lifestyles with cancer, showing that there is a strong connection between good nutrition and good health. The National Cancer Institute is involved in a research program testing the effects of vitamin A, beta carotene, vitamins C and E, and selenium, among others, to see whether they have an impact on cancer.

What is the macrobiotic diet?

The macrobiotic diet has received a great deal of publicity as a cure for cancer. There are many variations on the original diet, which was extremely restrictive and consisted mainly of brown rice. Liquids, usually in the form of miso or tamari broths, are used sparingly. Meat (including poultry), dairy products, tropical or semitropical fruits and juices, sugar, honey, and anything artificial are all avoided.

Can the macrobiotic diet be harmful to cancer patients?

The macrobiotic diet is lacking in nutritional elements needed by even healthy individuals. It is low in many vitamins and minerals. Since milk products are excluded, getting enough calcium can be a problem. For cancer patients, there are additional difficulties. Many are already experiencing weight loss and lack of appetite. People on the macrobiotic diet need to eat large amounts of food, mostly bulky foods, to obtain the number of calories required by the diet. The diet does not allow vitamin and mineral supplements.

What is known about what lifestyle habits cause cancer?

One major finding is that about 80 percent of cancers are linked to the way we live. Cigarette smoking contributes to at least 30 percent of all cancer deaths each year in the United States. While the relationship to diet is not as precisely defined, data increasingly point to the fact that diet plays a role in about 30 percent of all cancers, such as breast and colon cancers. Alcohol-related cancers are responsible for about 3 percent of deaths, viruses account for 5 percent, occupational exposures for at least 4 percent, and excessive sun exposure for about 3 percent.

What are the basic guidelines for cancer prevention?

Both the National Cancer Institute and the American Cancer Society suggest the following:
- Don't smoke or use tobacco in any form.
- Eat foods low in fat.
- Eat more foods that are high in fiber, such as whole grain cereals, fruits, and vegetables.
- Include foods rich in vitamins A and C in your daily diet.
- Watch your weight. People who are 40 percent or more overweight increase their risk of several kinds of cancer.
- If you drink alcoholic beverages, do so only in moderation.
- Avoid too much sunlight. Wear protective clothing.
- Use sunscreens.

How can I increase vitamins in the foods I eat?

Many vegetables and fruits contain vitamin A and C and beta carotene—vitamins proven to be effective in preventing cancer. The vitamin-rich dark green leafy vegetables, the red, yellow, and orange vegetables and fruits, citrus fruits and juices made from any of these are particularly good choices. Vegetables from the cabbage family, sometimes referred to as cruciferous vegetables, also may reduce cancer risk. Such vegetables as bok choy, broccoli, Brussels sprouts, cabbage, cauliflower, collards, kale, kohlrabi, mustard greens, rutabagas, and turnips and their greens are good choices. Remember that overcooking vegetables causes them to lose nutritional value. Eating a variety of fruits and vegetables is a good way to increase your vitamin intake.

Once treatments are completed and I'm back to normal, what should I remember about reducing fat in my diet?

Studies of populations in many countries around the world show that, almost without exception, the more fat consumed by a particular group of people, the higher the rate of cancer in that population. Studies of migrating populations indicate that the difference in cancer risk among nations cannot be entirely genetic but must be related to environmental factors. Evidence is growing that eating too much fat, both saturated and unsaturated, may increase your chances of getting cancers of the colon, breast, prostate, and endometrium. Reducing fat in the diet may reduce your cancer risk. And, at the same time, it can also control your weight and reduce your risk of heart attacks and strokes. During World War II in England and Wales, there was a drastic decrease in the amount of meat, fat, and sugar in the diet, and an increase in the amount of cereal and vegetables. There was also a marked reduction in deaths due to cancers of the breast and colon. In the years following the war, when fats in the diet were increased and fiber decreased, deaths from colon and breast cancer increased. According to the National Cancer Institute, the typical American diet consists of about 40 percent fat. Experts advise that the amount of total fat in the diet should be reduced to 30 percent.

How do I go about lowering the amount of fat in my diet?

It isn't easy—but once you learn how, you'll wonder how you ever could eat as much fat as you did. Here are some thoughts:

- Choose lean cuts of beef, lamb, and pork. Trim away as much of the fat before cooking as possible and trim again before eating.
- Choose chicken and turkey and remove skin and visible fat before cooking.
- Choose fresh fish and shellfish, plain frozen seafoods without sauce, and canned fish packed in water rather than canned fish packed in oil or fried seafood.
- If you use luncheon and variety meats, choose those that are labeled "reduced fat content."
- Dried peas and beans are less fatty than nuts and seeds.
- Snack on fresh or frozen fruits and vegetables and air-popped popcorn rather than pastries or deep-fried foods.
- Eat more fruits and vegetables, most of which are low in fat—with the exception of olives, avocados, coconut, and nuts. Be particularly aware of the fact that coconut oil turns up in a great variety of sweet foods, such as pastry products, as well as in granola-type cereals and nondairy substitutes.
- Choose low-fat dairy products more often than those made with whole milk or cream.
- Choose reduced-calorie or low-fat salad dressings and margarines.
- Use cooking methods that add little or no fat to foods.
- Broil, poach, or roast meats, and cook meats on racks so that fats are drained. Drain fat from pan before making gravy.
- Season vegetables with herbs, spices, and lemon juice rather than with fats and salt.

Why is fiber so important to good health?

Fiber contributes bulk or roughage to the diet and helps promote regular bowel movements. According to the National Cancer Institute, a diet high in fiber and low in fat may reduce the risk of cancers of the colon and rectum since it helps move food through the intestines and out of the body, promoting a healthy digestive tract.

What kinds of studies are there to show the importance of fiber in cancer prevention?

Studies have accumulated over the years which point to the importance of fiber in the diet. In 1983, a study by National Cancer Institute scientists done in two counties of eastern Nebraska looked at patients with colon and rectal cancer who had been diagnosed from 1970 to 1977 and a similar group of people who had not had cancer. They were interviewed for medical history, ethnic background, residence, diet, smoking, and occupation. Study findings showed there was an increase of colon cancer risk in those who ate a high-fat diet, particularly those whose diets were high in meat, dairy products, and sweets. Another study comparing Finnish and Danish population groups, which have similar dietary intakes of fat, found colon cancer incidence was much lower among the rural Finns, whose diet contains large amounts of high-fiber, unrefined rye bread, than among the Danes in Copenhagen, who have a low-fiber diet. However, the Cancer Institute is presently conducting further studies since most of the studies done in the past have been broad and have not assessed the specific components of fiber. These new studies will give more specific data.

How is fiber protective against colon-rectal cancer?

It is thought that fiber protects by hastening the travel time of fecal material through the bowel so that carcinogens are in contact with the bowel for a shorter period of time. In addition, the increase in the bulk of the stool may dilute the concentration of carcinogens, as well as changing the kinds of bacteria in the bowel.

How much fiber should I eat daily?

Most Americans get only about 11 grams of fiber daily. The National Cancer Institute recommends a total of 20 to 30 grams daily but no more than 35 grams.

How can I get more fiber into my daily diet?

Concentrate on foods made with whole grains and whole grain flour rather than those made with refined flour. Add bran and oatmeal. Eat more fruits and vegetables, both fresh and frozen. Apples, peaches, pears, and potatoes with their skins, as well as strawberries and raspberries, are good fiber sources. Cooked dry beans and peas are excellent sources. Foods that are high in fiber are usually filling and low in fat.

Are there studies that show a connection between fat and fiber?

There are some international studies of human populations which show that fiber may offer protection from the effects of fat. The problem is that which types of fiber are most effective and how they work is not fully known. In one animal study, rats were fed one of five diets containing various amounts of fat and fiber. The incidence and number of tumors per animal increased in all the fat-fed groups. Adding fiber to the diets provided partial protection against polyunsaturated fat and gave complete protection against saturated fat.

How can I tell if I am getting enough fiber in my diet?

One way of telling is to check your stools. If you are getting enough fiber in your diet, your stools will be large, soft, and easily passed without straining. The stools will float and will probably be about 4 or 5 inches long.

Are overweight people at higher risk for cancer?

A long-term study by the American Cancer Society among 750,000 men and women from 25 states and from all walks of life showed that individuals who were 40 percent or more overweight had a greatly increased risk of dying of cancer—55 percent higher for women and 33 percent higher for men. An average weight for all participants was determined for each sex and age group and for each inch of height. There were several cancer sites in which overweight people seemed to be especially susceptible. Women who were more than 40 percent overweight were five times more likely to have cancer of the endometrium (the inner lining of the uterus) than those of average weight. Rates for cancer of the uterus, gall bladder, and cervix were also four, three, and two times higher, respectively. Breast cancer was consistently higher for those overweight, increasing about one and a half times over women of average weight. In overweight men, rates were higher for colorectal and prostate cancers.

Are new studies being conducted on vitamins as they relate to colon cancer?

There has been mounting evidence on the effectiveness of vitamins in helping prevent colon cancer. One of the first studies, published in 1974, showed that both American and Norwegian patients with cancer of the digestive tract had less vitamin A in their diets than people who did not have these cancers. New studies are under way to try to refine and verify the effectiveness of a number of vitamins in relation to colon cancer. The effect of taking vitamin C and vitamin E alone or combined with wheat fiber on precancerous rectal growths is being tested in a New York City research study in patients who have previously undergone colorectal surgery. At the University of Chicago, people with low amounts of vitamin A in their diets or in their blood are being studied to see if they have an increased risk of colon polyps and/or colon cancer. Twelve hundred patients are being given daily supplements of beta carotene and/or vitamins C and E to see if either can prevent colon polyps in people at high risk in a study being conducted at Dartmouth College.

Is vitamin research being done in relation to cervical cancer?

Studies to see if forms of vitamin A (retinoids) will prevent or delay the beginning of cervical cancer in women who have abnormal cervical cells (diagnosed as moderate or severe dysplasia) and are at high risk of developing cervical cancer are now in progress. Three hundred women with this condition are being given the vitamin A retinoid in cream form for use with a collagen sponge within a cervical cap.

Are there vitamin studies being done concerning cancer of the esophagus?

A combination of 26 vitamins and minerals are being tested on 3,500 Chinese men and women who have abnormal cells in their esophagus (confirmed by microscopic examinations). There are approximately three new cases of esophageal cancers diagnosed each day among the 700,000 people in one rural county in China. This compares with one new case each month among whites in a comparable United States population. Half the group in the study will be given the vitamin supplements while the other half will be given a placebo that looks like the vitamin pill. Another Chinese group study being conducted in conjunction with the American National Cancer Institute involves 35,000 men and women in China who will be given a total of nine vitamins and minerals in four different combinations. Vitamin A, beta carotene, and zinc; riboflavin and niacin; vitamin C and molybdenum (a trace element); and selenium and vitamin E are the four groups being tested.

What studies are being done to determine if vitamins help prevent lung cancer?

A number of studies in various parts of this country and the world are under way. In Seattle, Washington, the Fred Hutchinson Cancer Research Center is recruiting persons occupationally exposed to asbestos who are at high risk for lung cancer and mesothelioma for a study of the cancer prevention effect of daily oral beta carotene and retinol (vitamin A). Another study at the same center involves smokers and ex-smokers. Twelve to fifteen thousand people will receive either some form of vitamin A plus beta carotene or a placebo. The study groups will be monitored for occurrence of lung cancer. Another group in Finland, which involves

20,000 male smokers, will compare the effect of oral synthetic beta carotene and vitamin E, separately and in combination, versus a placebo in reducing cases of lung cancer.

At the University of Alabama, 200 men who have smoked at least one pack of cigarettes a day for 20 years and have an abnormal sputum smear will be studied to see whether vitamin B12 and folate (folic acid, another B supplement) will reduce cases of lung cancer. In collaboration with the United Steel Workers of America, the University of Pittsburgh is studying 20,000 males who smoke one or more packs a day to see if the addition of beta carotene to their diet will reduce their risk for lung cancer and other diseases. The University of Texas Health Center is conducting a study of 350 men who were exposed to asbestos and 50 hospital patients with abnormal sputum tests to see if retinol and beta carotene will help prevent lung cancers.

Vitamin Supplements

If I decide to add vitamin/mineral supplements to my diet, what should I be aware of?

You should be informed about the levels of vitamins suggested by conservative physicians, based on the U.S. Recommended Dietary Allowance (RDA). You should understand that there are dosage levels for each individual vitamin that may produce toxicity or side effects. Additionally, you should inform your doctor that you are taking vitamin supplements. Certain vitamins interfere with the action of some medications and some test results may be altered by extra vitamin supplements in your system. Don't take vitamins haphazardly. Know what you are taking. It is important to take vitamins and minerals in combinations that work together. If you take only B5, for example, it may deplete your body's supply of other vitamins. Excess vitamin C can be responsible for the formation of kidney stones. Vitamins should be considered as supplements to a healthy, varied, nutritious diet.

There is no magic pill that can substitute for a full range of nutrients from a well-balanced diet.

What is the Recommended Dietary Allowance (RDA) of vitamins and minerals?

Commonly known as the RDA, it is the official guideline for the average daily amounts of nutrients that people should consume, based on an intake of about 2,000 calories a day. It provides nutrient guidelines in amounts sufficient to prevent well-known deficiency conditions such as scurvy, beriberi, and pellagra—but not necessarily to promote optimum health. Naturally, it does not take into account variations in individual needs or individual eating patterns. In preparing suggested diets below 1,600 calories daily, the Department of Agriculture found it impossible to assure RDA levels of all essential nutrients. Since about half of all American women consume fewer than 1,500 calories a day, it is almost a certainty that many are significantly deficient in many essential nutrients.

Which vitamins are most important in enhancing the immune system?

The vitamins that appear to play the greatest role in strengthening the immune system are beta carotene, B1, B5 (pantothenic acid), B6, and C. Zinc, a mineral, is also important.

Are megadoses of vitamins a good substitute for those who don't get enough vitamins from food?

Care must always be taken in adding vitamin supplements to the diet. In many cases, megadose vitamin therapy has been irresponsibly or even fraudulently touted, promising help it cannot deliver. This has overshadowed megavitamin therapy in general, but current research is under way in many medical centers to determine if high-dose vitamins can be helpful in preventing cancer. Though we don't mean to belabor the point, the best way to obtain the necessary vitamins is by eating a wide variety of foods. A multivitamin supplement is a safe hedge against deficiency. Most experts agree that it's safe to take a supplement containing up to twice the RDAs. What should be avoided, unless under a doctor's or qualified nutritionist's prescription, is self-megadosing. Megadosing is defined as taking 10 times the RDA for water-soluble vitamins and five times the RDA for fat-soluble vitamins. Taken in megadose quantities, some vitamins can be toxic and cause unpleasant and possibly dangerous side effects.

What's the difference between fat-soluble and water-soluble vitamins?

Fat-soluble vitamins are stored in the body's fat—so they do not necessarily have to be consumed every day. Water-soluble vitamins must be consumed daily in adequate amounts to meet the daily need, since they are continually being washed out of the body with urine and perspiration.

Which vitamins are fat-soluble?

A, D, E, and K are fat-soluble vitamins. Because they are stored in the body, there is danger of overdosing with fat-soluble vitamins, so caution must be used.

What are the water-soluble vitamins?

The eight B-complex vitamins and vitamin C are all water-soluble. Large percentages of these vitamins are lost during food processing, preparation, and storage. Often the water in which vegetables have been cooked contains more vitamins than remain in the cooked vegetables.

How does vitamin A affect the body?

Vitamin A is a powerful immune system stimulant. It has been shown to increase the size of the thymus gland, one of the important components of the immune system. Vitamin A can prevent the decrease in the size of the thymus that normally occurs after injuries. It has been used to decrease the development of cancer in animals exposed to cancer-causing chemicals. Vitamin A works better when it is taken with a zinc supplement.

Can vitamin A prevent cancer?

A growing number of laboratory and human studies indicate that there may be a connection between vitamin A and cancer prevention. About 20 studies undertaken in various parts of the world suggest that eating foods containing vitamin A might reduce the risk of developing cancer by some 30 to 50 percent. For instance, several controlled studies show lower vegetable consumption or lower estimates of vitamin A intake among patients with cancer than among controls. Three of these studied large groups—one of 8,278 Norwegian men, another of 265,118 Japanese adults, and the third of 2,107 American men—and found a lowered risk of lung cancer among those who ate food containing vitamin A. The Norwegian study showed that male smokers who consumed low amounts of vitamin A had a somewhat higher risk of lung cancer than those who consumed adequate amounts. Carrots, milk, and eggs were the main source of vitamin A in the men studied. The Japanese study, originally begun in 1965, was recently updated and expanded. The development of cancer was documented over a 10-year period. Daily consumption of vegetables high in beta carotene was linked with a decreased risk of developing cancers of the lung, colon, stomach, prostate, and cervix. There is evidence as well from the American study that the benefit may be related more to eating foods with beta carotene than to the vitamin A itself.

What is beta carotene and what is its relationship to vitamin A?

Beta carotene is a common source of vitamin A and is found in leafy green and yellow vegetables, certain fruits, liver, and dairy products. The beta carotene found in leafy green and yellow vegetables is converted to vitamin A in the digestive system. It is uncertain whether beta carotene's assocation with reduced cancer risk is due only to its conversion to vitamin A or whether beta carotene has some protective effect of its own. Many studies have reported a relationship between low risk for cancer and high consumption of foods containing beta carotene.

What are the most popular sources of beta carotene?

Carrots account for the major source of beta carotene in the diets of Americans. In Japan, yellow and green vegetables provide the major source of this important fat-soluble vitamin. In West Africa, red palm oil is the most important source of beta carotene. Large daily doses of natural beta carotene appear to be harmless and the body appears to convert to vitamin A only what it requires, so there should be no fear of developing vitamin A toxicity from an overdose of carrots.

Are retinoids also vitamin A?

Retinoids are derivatives and chemical cousins of vitamin A. Several animal studies have shown that vitamin A and the retinoids can prevent and reverse chemically induced lung tumors. However, natural retinoids are known to have toxic effects in animals, particularly at high doses. Researchers are now trying to develop synthetic retinoids that are as effective as natural retinoids in preventing cancer growth, but are less toxic and more specific to different cancer sites. One of these is 4-HPR.

What do tests of 4-HPR show?

This new, synthetic retinoid (4-hydro xyphenyl retinamide) has been shown to prevent the development of breast cancer in rats and bladder cancer in mice. Testing of 4-HPR in Italy has shown that it is less toxic than the standard retinoids such as vitamin A or the retinoic acids. Twenty-five hundred Italian women who have had breast cancer surgery, but were found to have no metastases, are being given 4-HPR to see if this substance will prevent new breast cancers from developing. The incidence of second breast cancers will be compared to 2,500 other breast cancer surgery patients who will receive a placebo.

Is vitamin A being used to prevent skin cancer?

A number of studies are assessing vitamin A in relation to skin cancer. A study at Memorial Sloan-Kettering Cancer Center in New York City is investigating whether beta carotene, or a combination of beta carotene and vitamins C and E, given to individuals at high risk for basal-cell skin cancer, may reduce the occurrence of new tumors. Also being studied is the role of the immune system and heredity in basal-cell skin cancer and the influence of beta carotene and a combination of beta carotene with vitamins C and E on immunity. At the National Cancer Institute, 13-cis-retinoic acid, a synthetic retinoid, is being given to 1,200 patients who have had two or more basal-cell carcinomas in the past five years to see if this retinoid will prevent a recurrence. Patients with basal-cell and squamous-cell skin cancers are being given beta carotene or a placebo in another study done under the auspices of Dartmouth College in which 1,950 patients are enrolled.

What are the B-complex vitamins?

The B vitamins are a family of vitamins that includes B1 (thiamine), B2 (riboflavin), B3 (niacin), B6 (pyridoxine), and B12 (cobalamin). The B vitamins are water-soluble, therefore you need them every day.

Are the B vitamins interdependent on one another?

Yes. The excess intake of any one may create a greater need for the others. Although most excess B vitamins are excreted in the urine, it is important to be aware of the dependence of one B vitamin on the others. Most of the low-dosage B complex supplements on the market have been properly balanced. Megadosages should be scrutinized because overdoses of one B vitamin, without the supplementation of the others, may throw the interrelationship off balance, resulting in deficiencies of the others. Several of the B vitamins are important to carbohydrate metabolism, so the more sugars and starches in your diet, the more B vitamins you probably need. B vitamins also can be washed out of your body by drinking a lot of coffee, tea, or alcohol, or by perspiring heavily.

Is there evidence that the B vitamins are involved in cancer prevention?

As early as 1944, scientists were investigating the potential of folic acid, a B vitamin, to retard the development of cancer. More recently, scientists have shown that folic acid (folate) plays a key role in how normal cells differentiate. Oral folic acid or a placebo, in this case vitamin C, was given daily for three months to 47 women with mild or moderate cervical dysplasia who were using combination-type oral contraceptives. Significant improvement was shown in the tissue slides of the folic acid-treated group compared to the vitamin C group, which showed no change. This suggests that the folic acid may prevent the progression of precancerous lesions and in some cases may promote them to reverse to normal. At the Cancer Center in Seattle, a detailed study of the effect of oral folic acid is being conducted with women at high risk of developing cervical cancer because they have mild to moderate cervical dysplasia. The women are receiving daily folic acid or a similar-appearing placebo, and are being examined every three months for a minimum of 12 months to determine whether their dysplasia has regressed or progressed. All patients are also having blood samples analyzed for serum folate, vitamin A, beta carotene, vitamin C, vitamin E, and for antibody levels for sexually transmitted organisms. Gynecological history, dietary and vitamin intake, and personal habits will also be included in the study.

Is niacin (vitamin B3) an important vitamin in preventing cell damage?

Niacin is essential to every cell in the body. Scientists have been able to show in laboratory dish experiments that niacin-deficient cells can be converted from normal to cancerous cells at a rate 10 times greater than normal cells. A deficiency of niacin may result when B6 is inadequate, because niacin cannot be produced properly when levels of B6 are low.

What role does vitamin C play in the body?

Vitamin C stimulates the immune system so that resistance to disease is improved. It is needed to protect the brain and spinal cord, for collagen syntheses, to manufacture neurotransmitters, and for lipid and carbohydrate metabolism. It is an antioxidant. We know that it is an essential substance, but it is not yet understood exactly how it works in the body. Its most obvious role is in the manufacture of collagen, the major component of skin, tendons, and bones. Vitamin C is believed to be most effective in the presence of B complex, E, and bioflavinoids. Overdosing can distort some test results, cause kidney stone formation and excess acidity. It has been proven that vitamin C inhibits the formation of nitrosamines, which have been shown to cause cancer in certain animals. Many commercial bacons and hot dogs are now processed with a form of vitamin C to help decrease the level of nitrosamines in the product.

Are there studies being done on vitamin C and cancer prevention?

Laboratory and animal research shows that vitamin C as well as vitamin E block the formation of nitrosamines, potential cancer-causing agents resulting from reactions in the digestive tract to nitrates, nitrites, and other substances added to foods. In some studies, large doses of vitamin C have completely protected rats against chemically induced kidney tumors. Other studies have shown that oral vitamin C was capable of blocking the formation of bladder tumors induced by implanted tablets of a chemical with cancer-causing potential. It is believed that vitamin C prevented the oxidation of the chemical from a potential to an actual carcinogen. In tissue-culture studies, vitamin C appears to prevent or reverse chemically induced cancer.

Another piece of evidence seems to come from the observation that Japanese men and women who migrated to Hawaii from areas where there is a high incidence of stomach cancer had Hawaiian-born children who showed a lowered risk for stomach cancer. Scientists hypothesize that the Hawaiian diet, including fruits and vegetables rich in vitamin C, may have contributed to this lowered risk. Since the diets in many of these studies contain not only vitamin C but also vitamin A, folic acid, and fiber, it is not clear which gives the protective effect.

Another study by a Canadian group found in examining

bowel movements that some people produce an agent, known as a mutagen, that alters genes. There is a close relationship between mutagens and carcinogens, and researchers suggest that this mutagen may possibly cause cancerous changes in the colon. Supplemental vitamin C plus vitamin E have been shown to reduce mutagen production. It is thought that these vitamins might be helpful in preventing colon cancer in persons at high risk. Studies are continuing, using vitamins C and E in persons who are at high risk for colon cancer.

Is there a connection between cancer, vitamin D, and calcium?

Drs. Cedric and Frank Garland have attempted to establish a link between a deficiency of vitamin D and calcium and cancers of the breast and colon. These doctors believe that when a lack of calcium occurs, the chemical code through which cells communicate is broken, signaling to the remaining cell that it should divide—thus causing cells to divide unnecessarily—physical evidence of a breakdown in the normal order of tissue formation. A book entitled *The Calcium Connection* by Cedric Garland (Putnam Publishing Group, 1988) shows how to determine how much calcium an individual needs based on sunlight, pollution, and water in the area where he lives and the foods he eats. The Garlands' studies seem to indicate that calcium absorption is profoundly affected by the level of vitamin D in the body. Because vitamin D is produced primarily by exposure to sunlight, where you live and how you live affect vitamin D levels. Their studies were prompted by findings of geographic health patterns, relating them to sunlight, vitamin D, and calcium. They used a nutritional study which had followed 1,954 men who worked at a Western Electric Plant near Chicago for 19 years. At the end of the period, 49 of the men had developed intestinal cancer; 1,372 were free of cancer. Analysis showed that those who developed cancer ate far fewer foods containing vitamin D and calcium. Men who took in the lowest amount of calcium had more than three times as much intestinal cancer as men who had the highest intake.

A study at Memorial Sloan-Kettering Cancer Center in New York City has focused on people at high risk of intestinal cancer because of a strong family tendency to develop the disease. The study was designed to see what effect calcium might have on the tissue of the intestinal tracts of these people. Before taking calcium, these high-risk people had an unusually high rate of cell division in the intestine. During the test they were given a dose of 1,250 milligrams of calcium carbonate per day. After several months of taking the dietary supplement, their intestinal cells stopped dividing at the abnormally high rate and began to divide at a rate typical of people at ordinary risk for intestinal cancer. In coming to their original conclusions, one exception to their general findings continued to puzzle the investigators. After all the data had been gathered, they were still baffled by the fact that Japanese women, who live in a region with only moderate sunlight, had a rate of breast and intestinal cancer of about five in 100,000. By comparison, other areas at the same latitude, such as San Francisco and Connecticut, have rates more than five times as high. The Garlands theorize that the missing link was that although Japanese women are not exposed to a great deal of sunlight, their diet provides the vitamin D their bodies need to help absorb calcium, and thus prevent breast and colon cancer. Research is continuing to try to confirm these findings.

What part does vitamin E play in the body?

Vitamin E is an antioxidant. It prevents the oxidation of fats, which is to say that it keeps fats from turning rancid by protecting lipids from the attack of oxidizing agents. You can appreciate the importance of vitamin E when you learn that all the cells of the body—brain cells, blood cells, muscle cells, nerve cells—are largely made up of membranes, which are made up of lipids. Vitamin E, also known as alpha-tocopherol, is found in vegetable oils, whole grains, liver, beans, fruits, and vegetables.

How does vitamin E react in the body?

Vitamin E, along with vitamin C, appears to prevent the formation of nitrosamines, potential cancer-causing agents that result from reactions in the human digestive system of substances readily found in food. Nitrites—which include nitrite salts added to meat for color, flavor development, and control of bacterial contamination; nitrate salts used in food processing that are reduced to nitrite in the body; and nitrogen oxides derived from the "smoking" process—react with amines and amides in the digestive tract to form nitrosamines and nitrosamides. Formentation processes, such as pickling and brewing, permit conversion of a variety of nitrogen sources, including ammonia and amino acids, to nitrite. Vitamins E and C compete in the body with the amine or amide for the nitrosating agent. If the vitamin "wins," reacting with the nitrosating agent, the formation of nitrosamines and nitrosamides is blocked.

What research is being done with vitamin E and cancer?

Researchers at the Johns Hopkins School of Hygiene and Public Health have reported an association between low-serum vitamin E levels and lung cancer risks. The scientists analyzed the blood of 99 people diagnosed with lung cancer along with the blood from 99 normal people; they found that the lung cancer risk of those with the lowest vitamin E level was 2.5 times greater than those with the highest vitamin E level. Vitamin E has also been reported to reduce the incidence of chemically induced tumors of the colon in mice.

Are trace minerals important?

The trace minerals are absolutely vital to the body's healthy operation and we are expanding our knowledge about the many trace elements with each passing year. Still, because both epidemiologic and animal studies regarding zinc and other trace metals such as copper, molybdenum, and iodine are limited, the connection between dietary and nutritional status and the functioning of the immune system has not been fully explored and documented. The close, and some- times completely opposite, conclusions of the relationships between zinc and iron, zinc and copper, as well as the in- volvement and interactions of selenium, cadmium, and other trace elements, indicate that there is still a great deal of mys- tery involved with the study of trace minerals, immune func- tion, and immune disease. The absorption of minerals into the bloodstream is a highly variable process, influenced by many factors. Pregnant women, for example, absorb calcium much more efficiently than others, and iron is absorbed much better if it is taken along with an acid food such as orange juice. Overdosing with iron supplements can cause accidental poisoning in children. Depriving the body of io- dine can produce mental and physical retardation in children and a variety of serious health problems in adults.

What does selenium do?

Selinium forms a part of large enzyme molecules. Its primary role is as an antioxidant, preventing breakdown of fats and other body chemicals. It is known to interact with vitamin E. Studies have shown that people who live in areas where se- lenium levels are low in water and soil have higher cancer rates and show more deaths from high blood pressure. A study in mice shows that when selenium is added to drinking water, the incidence of breast cancer and precancerous tumors such as colon cancer is reduced. Given to animals before the development of cancer cells by viral or chemical means, selenium appears to prevent the onset of cancer. It must be noted, however, that selenium has not succeeded in inhibiting the growth rate of tumors that were already established. Selenium is an essential element in the body. However, as is the case with many essential elements, it is harmful when taken at high levels. Selenium is found in seafoods, organ meats, onions, and grains, especially those grown in some selenium-rich areas.

How does zinc relate to selenium?

Animal studies have shown that if 200 parts per million of zinc are available in water, small amounts of selenium uptake are prevented in the face of these high zinc levels. It is theorized that high levels of zinc can block the effects of selenium.

Are there any studies that show whether or not selenium might prevent cancer?

There are both laboratory and animal studies which show that certain forms of selenium may possibly prevent cancer. A Columbia University study has reported that selenium may "protect" against radiation- and chemically induced cancer in cells grown in the laboratory. Many animal experiments have shown that it may have a protective effect. There are also epidemiologic studies from a number of geographical areas that show higher cancer risks when there is less selenium concentrated in the water supply or soil or in blood levels. In the northeastern United States there are high colon, rectal, and breast cancer rates. Researchers feel they are correlated with industrialization, diets high in fat, and a low amount of selenium in the soil. According to the National Cancer Institute, in most areas studied, where selenium level is low, some cancer rates are high. However, whether this is a cause-effect relationship cannot be accurately established because of other effects such as industrialization and diet differences. Moreover, it is not clear whether this relationship applies to all types of cancer or only to specific ones, such as cancers of the digestive tract. Data related to selenium intake are being gathered now in studies in China, Finland, and other countries where people are receiving selenium supplements or have low selenium intakes. In addition, the National Cancer Institute is funding several studies on selenium.

What kinds of studies are being done by the National Cancer Institute on selenium?

The National Cancer Institute and the U.S. Department of Agriculture have begun collaborative studies to determine the body's response to, dietary assessment of, interactions of, and measurements of selenium. There are three ongoing studies. In the first, healthy volunteers received a single dose of both organic and inorganic selenium. The researchers are examining body responses to both forms. The other two studies are designed to determine a range of acceptable dose levels and chemical forms of selenium suitable for use in human cancer prevention trials. The first study is being conducted with 90 healthy volunteers in South Dakota, where the highest selenium intake in the United States occurs; the second is being done with several hundred normal volunteers in a county in China, which, in the past, reported cases of selenium intoxication, resulting from the fact that daily selenium levels there are 20 times higher than the upper limits generally considered acceptable in the United States.

What are free radicals and antioxidants?

Free radicals are by-products of normal chemical reactions in your body that can make a cell develop into cancer if not destroyed. Free radicals are also increased by harmful chemicals known to cause cancer. However, the body has natural protection against free radicals thanks to certain vitamins and minerals known as antioxidants, which serve as free radical scavengers. Beta carotene, vitamins A, C, and E, zinc, selenium, and copper are potent antioxidants.

How do free radicals alter cells?

Carcinogens such as X-rays and sunlight are associated with free radical reactions capable of altering the cell's DNA. These chemical changes in the DNA alter the cell's normal regulation and may be related to cancer development. Some chemical carcinogens enter the body in an active form. Others that are inactive when they enter may be converted into active forms by the normal processes of various organs or by combining with other chemicals in the digestive tract. For example, nitrates can combine in the stomach with amines to form nitrosamines or with amides to form nitrosamides. This does not take place when some antioxidants, especially vitamin C, are present. Animal studies have shown that agents such as beta carotene, vitamins A, C, E, and the trace element selenium may prevent, inhibit, or reverse carcinogenesis—possibly by blocking free radical reactions at the molecular level. Whether nitrosamines and nitrosamides are significant carcinogens in humans is still being debated.

What is known about our need for zinc?

Zinc is required for both DNA and RNA synthesis. Many studies show that a deficiency in zinc weakens the ability of thymidine to be incorporated into DNA and adversely affects all the steps that occur in reproducing cell population. Several enzymes involved in RNA and DNA synthesis seem to require zinc.

Have the effects of zinc been studied in healthy individuals?

Scientists in Brussels have conducted research showing that zinc supplementation may have a regulatory effect on the immune systems of normal, healthy individuals. Eighty-three persons, all healthy adults, young men, young and older women, some taking oral contraceptives, were given daily supplements of zinc. Another group of individuals was studied but not given the supplements. After a month of taking the zinc, all 83 persons in the zinc-taking group showed an increase in the response of lymphocyte cells of the immune system.

What foods are high in zinc?

Lobster and deep-sea fish have the highest amounts of zinc per milligram. Soy meal, wheat bran, black-eyed peas, crab and oysters, beef, lamb, dark turkey meat, and organ meats all show high levels of zinc. Zinc can also be supplied in pill or liquid form.

Why is potassium important to the body?

The main functions of potassium are in the maintenance of the body's water content, nerve conduction, and muscle contraction. It also triggers certain enzyme reactions and is concentrated within cells. Since the body cannot conserve its potassium efficiently, potassium deficiencies can set in quite easily as a result of diarrhea, fasting, excessive sweating, or the use of diuretic drugs. Potassium is readily available in foods such as dried apricots, prunes, raisins, bananas, molasses, and potatoes.

What research has been done on potassium intake and cancer?

According to a 10-year study done in Texas, high potassium intake can significantly decrease cancer risk. Noticing the low colon–rectal cancer rate in Seneca County, New York, though the area is located in a region with the highest colon–rectal cancer rate in the nation, studies were undertaken to determine what factors were involved. The researchers believe the unique geochemical makeup of Seneca County to be the most probable explanation for the low rate of colon–rectal cancer. Seneca's drinking water comes from two deep glacial lakes that penetrate the underlying salt strata, causing the sum of the concentrations of high potassium and low sodium to be between 10 and 20 times higher than that in other lakes in the state. In correlating information, researchers noted that the Great Salt Lake area in Utah has the lowest cancer rates in the United States. Potassium salt concentration in this lake was found to be even higher than in Seneca's lakes and the potassium/sodium ratio three times higher than that of the lakes at Seneca.

What vitamins can help to increase potassium levels?

Both vitamins A and C have been found to increase the intracellular potassium/sodium ratio. Low cancer rates have been associated with high-fiber vegetables and fruits, which are also high in potassium and low in sodium.

Are there known potassium depleters?

Vomiting, diarrhea, and the use of diuretics lower potassium levels. Licorice is known to deplete potassium levels—and since licorice is an additive widely used in tobacco products, it is believed that licorice may be a contributing factor in the high cancer rate among smokers.

What is co-enzyme Q10?

Co-enzyme Q10 is a naturally occurring nutrient that is part of every living cell. Scientists have found that Q10 is an integral part of the immune cycle. When immunity is low, so, it has been discovered, are the reserves of Q10. When Q10 is boosted, so is the immune potential. The drugs used in treating cancer do their job by killing off the cancerous cells, but they also knock out protective immune responses. Q10 appears to have the ability to assist in the production of antibodies, producing a significant reversal of the immunosuppression.

How can Q10 be added to the diet?

Mackerel and sardines contain the largest amounts of this co-enzyme. Spinach and broccoli are the two popular vegetables with the highest significant content. Supplemental Q10 is available over the counter; it can be taken at mealtimes and will digest naturally along with other foods. Since this co-enzyme has not been placed by the FDA in any drug classification, no health benefits can be claimed by the manufacturers. The FDA must review the claims and accept exhaustive studies that prove beneficial applications and lack of toxicity. Presently Q10 is available and marketed as a dietary supplement without health claims, though it has been used in Japan since the 1970s as a prescription drug. Medical researchers are investigating the effectiveness of Q10 on cancer patients who develop toxicity from long-term treatment with Adriamycin, which results in damage to the heart. This toxicity has been reported in 2 to 20 percent of patients receiving Adriamycin. Among the heart-healthy population, the risk factor from Adriamycin is only 2 percent, but among patients with underlying valvular, coronary, or myocardial disease, a history of hypertension, or people over age 70, the risk factor is much greater. It appears from some studies that patients who took Q10 along with Adriamycin were able to tolerate dosages of the drug with little or no changes in heart function.

chapter 6

The Days Ahead

Though at the time of diagnosis people say they can't think of a worse "rap," many people—too many for it to be coincidental—say that the cancer experience which had seemed so negative to them at the start turned out to be one of the most positive things that had ever happened to them. To those who haven't experienced it, this sounds bizarre. But upon examination we find that the awareness of life that the threat of cancer brings with it sharpens all the senses, strengthens bonds, matures the outlook, and focuses inner strengths.

Finding out you have cancer has been described as a feeling of moving between life and death, an awkward place to be. You've survived the hardest times, the period of moving blindly from one thought to another with nonstop images of fear and panic. You've come to the point where you can look at your life and can order your own priorities. You've learned to value life by quality not quantity. You've grown to understand the "chronic-ness" of cancer. You've learned that each of us must face death and accept it in our own way. The opportunity to "put your affairs in order" and do so in an orderly and organized manner is a major benefit that is mentioned by many people.

> *"I keep finding positive results of my illness. I
> probably have not completely overcome my
> cancer but have learned to live a normal life
> while continuing treatment. I continue normal
> activities as much as possible and do things I
> had wanted to do previously but* wouldn't.*"*
>
> *Diagnosed with leukemia in 1983 at age 44*

Following through with proper medical care makes good
sense for anyone—and especially for anyone who has had
cancer. It's assurance for the good health you have "bought"
for yourself. It is insurance that any chance of recurrence will
be dealt with immediately. Being aware of your body and all
its nuances is healthy, unless you swing in the opposite direction and worry yourself needlessly by suspecting every ache
and pain. Making constructive, health-assuring changes in
your lifestyle will result in a renewed affirmation of life.
Being aware and acting on the facts about smoking, fiber, fat,
stress, exercise, and vitamins are all positive ways of following through with your own care. It's true that your life will
never be the same as it was before. But the changes can be
enriching and rewarding. You, as have many others, may find
that your experience with cancer is responsible for developing unexpected spiritual and intellectual depths that allow
you to search and find new personal meanings, to view yourself and your life more critically and with new intensity and
appreciation. Knowing about your own cancer and understanding symptoms is an important factor in your continuing
health. Being aware of your checkup needs gives you added
confidence and protection.

**When I'm having treatments, what kind of side effects
should I let my doctor know about?**

There are a number of side effects that should alert you to
contact your doctor:

- Fever—with a temperature over 101 or a very low temperature (90).
- A very sore throat or mouth, or ulcers in the throat or mouth.
- Dizziness, lethargy, or shortness of breath.
- Profuse sweating or chills strong enough to cause shaking.
- A severe cold, cough, or flu. The doctor may decide to delay treatment because of it.
- Bruises or tiny bleeding spots on the skin.
- Severe nausea or vomiting.
- Severe constipation or diarrhea.
- Marked pain or inflammation where chemotherapy or radiation were given.
- Severe headaches or other severe pain.

Any and all of these symptoms are important to report to the physician as soon as possible.

Why am I terrified by every ache and pain?

This is a normal reaction. Many triumphers say that they have gone through the routine of thinking every cough, every bone ache, every headache, every change in regular health routine, was a sign that they had cancer again. To help put the whole experience in perspective, you should talk over your fears with your physician. Ask him for the facts on your type of cancer—what the chances are of recurrence, where metastases usually occur, and what symptoms you should watch for. Facts will help put your mind at rest so that you can concentrate your energies on enjoying your recovery and good health.

What kind of medical follow-up do I need after cancer treatment?

Most likely, you will return for checkups to the doctor who directed your case. This could be your medical oncologist, or depending on the treatment, site, and stage of your cancer, it could be your surgeon (as is often the case with breast cancer), a specialist (such as a urologist for prostate cancer), a radiation therapist, or a combination of several doctors. You should probably also be followed by your family doctor, who will be giving you routine care such as physicals, blood tests, Pap tests, and blood stool tests. Usually, during the first year you will see the cancer specialist every three months. During the second to fifth years your schedule will probably be changed to every six months; then appointments will gradually be reduced to a yearly schedule. Naturally each physician will tailor-make a follow-up for each patient, so the generalized information in this chapter which refers to follow-up care is simply a guideline, giving you a general idea of what to expect.

Though the last thing you probably want to do at this point is spend time in a doctor's office, follow-up care is a necessary part of your life and it is important that you stick to scheduled appointments. Be an active partner in the follow-up. Report promptly any new or persistent symptoms so that they may be evaluated by the physician—and so they can be removed from your "worry list" as quickly as possible. Life-long follow-up on a regular programmed schedule is important. Though it may make you feel anxious when you're anticipating it, when it's over, you'll feel immensely relieved and reassured.

"About checkups. I go, frequently. I'm only afraid when there is pain. Today I found that what I feared was bone metastasis was actually bursitis. The sooner it is diagnosed, the sooner it can be treated. Time is our enemy. Cancer survivors like me must be ever vigilant and on top of the situation. It's too easy to fall through the cracks with so many doctors. One must lead the team and take responsibility."

Diagnosed with lymphoma in 1984 at age 38

What kinds of tests will be done during checkups?

Usually the cancer specialist will ask specific questions, depending on your cancer, adding to your medical history. You'll have a chance to talk about any problems you have had since your last visit. A physical examination will be done, concentrating on the kind of cancer you had and the area of your treatment. Blood samples will be taken and chest X-rays may be needed. These are followed by tests that depend on your type and stage of cancer. There is no really firm agreement among doctors on which tests are needed and how often they should be done—but there are some general guidelines for suggested follow-up that may be helpful to you. Additional tests may be necessary, depending upon your doctor's advice, your history, or your symptoms, if any. Just having a general idea of what is normally required helps in putting your mind at ease about your checkup. We cover here the kinds and frequencies of various tests that may be ordered by your doctor for the more common kinds of cancers, in addition to taking a history, performing a yearly physical and doing the usual blood tests. The common "signal" symptoms you should discuss immediately with your doctor if they occur are also listed.

What kind of follow-up is made for bladder cancer?

Analysis of urine and kidney function is usually done every three months for the first year, every six months during the second to fifth year, and yearly thereafter. You will probably have a cystoscopy (an examination of the lining of the bladder) on the same schedule. IVP and chest X-rays may be done yearly or more often, depending on location of the operation.

Signal symptoms: blood in urine, painful or difficult urination or urinating more often than usual.

What is the checkup schedule for primary bone or soft-tissue sarcomas?

Children and adults with primary bone or soft-tissue sarcomas will be checked by their physicians every three months for the first two years, every four months during the third year, every six months in the fourth and fifth years, and yearly thereafter. Chest X-rays or computerized tomography (CT scans) will usually be done at each visit. Periodically, bone scans and blood and urine tests will be done.

Signal symptoms: pain, lumps, loss of appetite or weight, or difficulty in breathing.

How often will I need to see a physician following a brain tumor?

If you had a tumor of the brain, you will probably be asked to return to your doctor every three months for the first year, every six months for the second to fifth years, and yearly thereafter. CT scans or MRI will probably be done every six months for the first year and yearly thereafter; chest X-rays yearly.

Signal symptoms: headaches, mental changes, motor problems, speech or balance problems.

How often will I need to return for checkups following breast cancer?

The doctor will probably ask you to return at three-month intervals for the first year and every six months thereafter. He will probably do a bone scan every six months the first year; a chest X-ray every six months the first year and yearly thereafter; blood tests at three, six, and 12 months and a mammogram yearly.

Signal symptoms: bone or chest pain, weight or appetite loss, or persistent cough. The most crucial period is the first two years, but follow-up must continue for the rest of your life.

What is the usual checkup schedule when you've had cancer of the cervix, vagina, or vulva?

Your doctor will probably ask to see you every three months for the first year, every six months the second to fifth years, and yearly thereafter. Depending upon what surgery was done, a Pap test may be needed at every visit. You may have an intravenous pyelogram (IVP) or CT scan at the end of the first year and chest X-rays yearly; urine and stool tests every six months through the fifth year and then yearly.

Signal symptoms: vaginal discharge or bleeding, bone pain, weight or appetite loss, bowel or bladder problems, or swelling of the legs.

What tests should I expect to have when I go for checkups for colon-rectal cancer?

You will probably be scheduled for a visit every three months in the first two years and every six months thereafter. Carcinoembryonic antigen (CEA), as well as blood, urine, and blood stool tests, will probably be ordered at every visit. You may have a CT scan every six months, colonoscopy or barium enema every year, and a sigmoidoscopy every six months for the first two years and yearly thereafter.

Signal symptoms: appetite or weight loss, changes in bowel function or urine color, abdominal pain, or jaundice.

What follow-up procedures are suggested for cancer of the esophagus?

Follow-up is suggested every three months the first year, every four months the second to fifth years and then every six months. Chest X-rays and blood stool tests may be done at each visit. Barium swallow is suggested at three, six, and 12 months, and then yearly. CEA and urine tests may be done at six and 12 months and yearly thereafter.

Signal symptoms: chest pain, difficulty in swallowing, lumps, change in bowel habits, a cough or hoarseness, or appetite or weight loss.

Is careful follow-up critical for Hodgkin's disease?

Careful follow-up is needed. Regular visits are usually scheduled every month or two for the first year, then every three to six months for the next four years, and annually thereafter. Chest X-rays and blood tests are done at every visit and urine tests every year. At the end of the first year, CT scans of the chest and abdomen may be ordered.

Signal symptoms: fever, itching, alcohol-induced pain, night sweats, lumps, or breathing problems. The crucial period is the first five years; if disease-free after five years, you're probably cured.

What follow-up is recommended for non-Hodgkin's lymphoma?

Suggested follow-up is every three months for the first year, every four months for the second to the fifth years, then yearly thereafter. Chest X-rays and blood tests are suggested at every visit; urine tests every year and ultrasound or CT scans of the abdomen and pelvis every year.

Signal symptoms: appetite or weight loss, fever, pain, lumps, difficulty in breathing, intestinal symptoms, or personality or balance problems.

What's the usual follow-up for kidney cancer?

You'll probably be seen every three months for the first year, every four months for the next four years, and then every year. Blood and urine tests will be done at every visit. Chest X-rays are suggested at three, six and 12 months and then every year; ultrasound or CT scans at six and 12 months and then yearly.

Signal symptoms: painful or bloody urination, respiratory or back or bone pain, weight loss, fatigue or loss of appetite, personality changes, or balance problems. The crucial period is the first three years, but follow-up should continue for life.

What follow-up is usually carried out for leukemia?

The follow-up depends upon the type of leukemia. For ALL, patients are seen monthly during maintenance chemotherapy, for blood work, with bone marrow checked yearly and chest X-rays and lumbar punctures done as needed. For CLL, you will probably be seen every four months for the first two years, then every year. Blood counts and other blood work will be done at every visit. Liver function tests, blood stool tests, other laboratory tests, chest X-rays, and liver spleen scans will be checked every year. If you have AML, you will be followed on a three-, six-, and 12-month schedule, then yearly. Blood, bone marrow, and other laboratory tests will be done. Liver function and urinary tests and chest X-rays are completed every year. Patients with CML will be seen at two-month intervals and then at six months, one year, and every two years. Blood counts and other blood work will be done along with uric acid tests. Bone marrow is checked at the two-year intervals.

Signal symptoms: fever, weight loss, bone pain, and night sweats.

What kind of follow-up is usually recommended for lung cancer?

Lung cancer patients are usually asked to come in for examination and chest X-rays once every three months the first year, once every four months the second through fifth year, and every six months from then on. Blood, urine, and CEA (and sputum cytology, if needed) will probably be checked at six and 12 months, then annually.

Signal symptoms: coughs, wheezing, labored breathing, loss of appetite or weight, chest or back pain, hoarseness, or any swelling of the face and arms.

"I deal poorly with checkups. They're a constant reminder that I'm sick. I call the doctor's office prior to an appointment to see if he's on time so I won't have to wait in the waiting room. I hate being in a room with people who only talk about cancer and illness."

Diagnosed with leukemia in 1986 at age 46

What is the suggested follow-up procedure for melanoma?

Follow-up will depend on the stage of the melanoma and the depth of involvement. Complete skin exams may be scheduled every two to four months for the first year, every four months for the next four years, then every six to 12 months.

Blood tests probably will be on the same schedule. Chest X-rays and liver tests will be done yearly.

Signal symptoms: changes in other spots on the skin, gastrointestinal problems, difficulty in breathing, unusual pain, lumps, personality changes, or balance problems. The crucial period is the first two years, with lifelong follow-up needed.

What kind of follow-up is suggested for ovarian cancer?

You'll probably be asked to return to the doctor every three months for the first year, every six months thereafter. Blood tests, Pap smears, urine tests, and tests for tumor markers may be done every six months; chest X-rays or CT scans yearly.

Signal symptoms: changes in abdominal size, pelvic pain, vaginal bleeding, masculinizing signs, or swelling of the legs.

What is the usual follow-up schedule for prostate cancer?

Most doctors will ask to see you every three months for the first year, every six months for the second through fifth years, and yearly thereafter. Urine, blood, and prostate specific antigen (PSA) tests will be done at checkups. Bone scans and chest X-rays may be ordered.

Signal symptoms: bone pain, urinary or cardiac symptoms.

What follow-up is needed for cancer of the stomach and small intestine?

The doctor will probably want to examine you every three months for the first two years, then every six months for the next three years, and annually thereafter. Blood and stool tests will be done at each of these visits. Liver function,

CEA, and CT scans may be done every six months, and chest X-rays and GI series on a yearly basis.

Signal symptoms: changes in abdominal size, pain in the abdomen, heartburn, nausea or vomiting, jaundice, difficulty in swallowing, and bowel-function changes.

What kind of follow-up is recommended for testicular cancer?

Meticulous follow-up with chest X-rays, blood tests, and tumor markers is recommended every three months during the first year, every four months for the next four years, and then yearly. CT scans of the abdomen are needed at six and 12 months, then yearly for two years.

Signal symptoms: abdominal pain, cough, leg swelling, appetite or weight loss, or respiratory problems. Critical period: nearly all patients who have completed therapy and are free of disease for four years can be considered cured.

How frequently should thyroid cancer be followed up?

Depending on the type of tumor, doctors see thyroid cancer patients every two to six months for the first five years, then yearly. Blood tests and chest X-rays are recommended at each visit. Thyroid scans will be done usually one month after treatment and may be done at the year-end mark.

Signal symptoms: cough, hoarseness, lumps, bone pain, and muscle spasms.

What kinds of tests are recommended following uterine (endometrium) cancer?

Examination by your physician will probably be done every three months the first two years, every four to six months the second through fifth year, and then yearly. Examination will probably include pelvic exam, stool, blood, tumor markers and urine tests, and Pap smear. Chest X-rays are done yearly.

Signal symptoms: any vaginal bleeding, pelvic pain, change in abdominal size, or swelling of the legs. The most crucial period is the first three years, but follow-up must continue.

Even though I am going back for my regular checkups for the cancer I had, should I still be following the recommendations of the American Cancer Society for regular physicals?

Being aware of the importance of finding cancer early, you can appreciate the need for keeping up to date on regular checkups for the parts of your body that are not being checked regularly during your cancer checkups. The following recommendations still hold for you, as they do for those who have never had cancer or who have no symptoms:

- Between the ages of 20 and 40, men should have a physical exam with health counseling and a cancer checkup every three years. This should include exams for cancer of the thyroid, testes, prostate, mouth, skin, and lymph nodes. Women should have a breast exam by a doctor every three years (in addition to doing a monthly breast self-exam), a mammogram between the ages of 35 and 40, and a Pap test every year after the age of 18. After three consecutive negative Pap tests, you should discuss with your doctor how often to have one. For young women who are under 18 and sexually active, regular Pap tests should be scheduled. Women aged 20 to 40 should also have a pelvic exam every three years and a physical with health counseling and cancer checkup every three years, including exams for cancer of the thyroid, mouth, ovaries, skin, and lymph nodes.
- After the age of 40, men should have a digital rectal exam every year, a physical exam with health counseling, and cancer checkup every year, including exams for cancer of

the thyroid, testes, prostate, mouth, skin, and lymph nodes. After 50, it is recommended that men should have a blood stool test every year and a proctosigmoidoscopy every three to five years following two consecutive negative exams.

Women over 40 should have a breast exam performed by a doctor every year in addition to monthly breast self-exams, a mammogram every one to two years between 40 and 49, and every year after 50. They should also have a pelvic exam, a physical with health counseling, and a cancer checkup every three years, including exams for cancers of the thyroid, mouth, ovaries, skin, and lymph nodes. Digital rectal exams as well as blood stool tests should be done each year. Pap tests should continue every three years (after two consecutive negative tests). Proctosigmoidoscopy is recommended every three to five years following two consecutive negative examinations. Endometrial tissue samples should be taken at menopause.

How can I keep track of whether or not my tests are up to date?

It is wise to keep a personal record of your tests, noting on your calendar when the next test is due. In this way, you can remind your doctor when it's time for your test even if he should overlook the need.

Guidelines by the American Cancer Society for Cancer Screenings In People Without Symptoms*		
Age 20–40	**Men** ✔Physical exam with health counseling and cancer checkup every three years, including exams for cancer of the thyroid, testes, prostate, mouth, skin, and lymph nodes	**Women** ✔Breast exam performed by a doctor every three years in addition to monthly breast self-exam

Age 20–40	Men	Women
		✔Pap test every year after age 18; following three consecutive negative tests discuss frequency with your doctor. If you are under 18 and sexually active, you should have regular Pap tests
		✔Pelvic exam every three years
		✔Physical with health counseling and cancer checkup every three years, including exams for cancers of the thyroid, mouth, ovaries, skin, and lymph nodes
Over 40	✔Digital rectal exam every year	✔Breast exam performed by a doctor every year, in addition to monthly breast self-exam
	✔Physical exam with health counseling and cancer checkup every year, including exams for cancer of the thyroid, testes, prostate, mouth, skin, and lymph nodes	✔Mammogram every one to two years between the ages of 40 and 49 and every year after age 50
	✔After age 50, a blood stool test every year, and a proctosigmoidoscopy every three to five years following two consecutive negative exams one year apart	✔After three annual consecutive negative Pap tests, discuss frequency with your doctor
		✔Pelvic exam every year
		✔Physical with health counseling and cancer checkup every three years, including exams for cancers of the thyroid, mouth, ovaries, skin, and lymph nodes
		✔Digital rectal exam every year
		✔After age 50, blood stool test every year and proctosigmoidoscopy every three to five years following two consecutive negative exams one year apart
		✔Endometrial tissue sample at menopause
	*People who are at higher risk for certain cancers may need tests more often	

Can the treatment I have had for cancer cause me to get a second cancer?

Some treatments which are very effective in fighting cancer may increase a person's risk of having another cancer later on. For example, high-energy radiation can cause bone cancer and certain chemotherapy drugs given at high doses can later cause leukemia. However, the risk of leukemia after treatment is estimated to be only 5 percent 10 years later. This risk seems highest in patients over 40 years old, who have been treated with intensive chemotherapy or with both chemotherapy and radiation therapy. When radiation alone is used, the rate of new cancer is far less than 1 percent. Generally, these patients were being treated for Hodgkin's disease or cancer of the ovary in cases where the disease would have been fatal if left untreated. In a study conducted by the National Cancer Institute of children who had survived cancer, researchers found a slightly increased risk of bone cancer in patients treated with chemotherapy and radiation therapy. Hodgkin's disease patients were also found to be twice as likely to develop cancer within five years after treatment as was the general population. Most of these patients had received radiation as part of their treatment.

Lung cancer was the most frequent cancer developed. However, all the persons who developed lung cancer were smokers. Because the number of lung tumors was greater than would be expected in the average smoking population, the researchers felt that radiation treatment might have increased the risk for lung cancer in these patients. Survivors should be aware that many of the things that increase the risk of cancer in the general population, such as smoking, may put them at even greater risk.

Will I ever get over the fear that cancer might be contagious?

That worry plagues many people—and it's understandable. When we don't know the cause of a disease, it is human nature to think that it might be contagious. Cancer has been with us a long time, but there is absolutely no true evidence that it is contagious. Certain viruses seem to be carcinogenic and cause cancer when they are injected into rats, monkeys, and dogs. But scientists say that this does not happen with humans. Family members living with or taking care of someone with cancer do not catch it. Doctors and nurses who care for cancer patients on a daily basis do not have a higher incidence of cancer than does the general population. There is no evidence to suggest that living in the same household with a cancer patient over a long period of time, sharing his or her possessions, kissing, drinking out of the same glass, or swimming in the same pool increases your chances of getting cancer.

Can I have a healthy baby even if I had cancer when I was a child?

Many of today's young adults who had cancer in their youth can look forward to having children without worrying that those children would be at high risk for developing cancer. In a study conducted by the National Cancer Institute in collaboration with scientists from five research centers around the country and involving nearly 2,300 survivors of childhood and adolescent cancers, it was found that most youths who survive cancer can later become parents without risk of their children getting cancer. A few children in the study did develop cancers that are known to be hereditary. Other than these, there was no evidence that the children of the long-term survivors developed cancer because their parent had it or because of their parent's cancer treatment.

Is it true that my relationship with my daughter can be affected for a long time after my breast cancer?

It appears from a number of studies that breast cancer is likely to have an emotional impact not only on you as a patient but on your children as well—and that daughters are more likely to have this problem than are sons. In addition, one study points out that when the breast cancer and treatment have been severe or prolonged, problems become more frequent. In one half the cases in this study, patients' relationships with their children remained much the same or were better than before. In many of these cases, greater closeness and understanding were noted. When relationships changed for the worse, the breast cancer patients tended to have a worse prognosis, difficulty in adjusting emotionally to cancer, and a more severe type of surgery. Relationships with adolescent and postadolescent daughters seemed to be the most vulnerable to difficulties. There is no question that a poor prognosis is frightening to everyone—especially children, causing them to withdraw from the mother. On the other hand, in cases where the cancer prognosis is not good, the mother may begin to withdraw from her children in response to or in anticipation of her worsening physical state.

In reflecting upon the meaning of this study, one obvious explanation for daughters' reactions is that daughters are placed at risk by a mother's breast cancer in a way that sons are not. Emotional upset and anger may result when the daughter reflects upon her own risk. In younger daughters, the fear may be focused on the threat to their mother's life at a time when they are still dependent upon her in the home. Another factor may be that mothers often lean more heavily on their daughters for support, thus creating demands that the daughters are unable to fulfill. When those needs are met, mother and daughter grow closer. If the daughter is unwilling or unable to provide this support, the mother's expectations are not fulfilled and conflict can result. Discussing the fears and talking about each one's needs can help to lessen the emotional stresses.

Something to Think About

- What things would I like to be able to say to those who mean the most to me?
- How do I feel as I think about saying those words?
- Do I have the courage to say them?
- What is the worst reaction I could get from them if I say them?
- Am I ready to say them?

ACTION: Write down your thoughts and practice what you want to say so you'll be able to express yourself when you feel the time is right (and the sooner the better).

Why do I find that hospitals and hospital smells make me anxious?

Certain studies have shown that some of the smells and other reminders of treatment can bring back the anxiety, even years after the treatment has finished. For instance, researchers have found that the sight of the hospital brought mild reactions in patients. For some, the smells in the clinic triggered a feeling of nausea and anxiety some 10 years after the treatment had ended. Most often the sights or smells brought back the same physical and emotional reactions felt during treatment.

Is it unusual for me to dream about the day I was diagnosed even though I completed my treatment more than five years ago?

Although the issues of survivors' problems have not been widely studied, there is some research that shows a small percentage of patients can have "flashback" experiences, especially in the first few years after treatment. These can happen in waking or sleeping hours. Some people show a difficulty in concentrating; others can't sleep; still others have recurring dreams. Unwanted thoughts and feelings can linger for years. Support groups are useful places to talk out these problems. If they persist, you may need to get professional help.

Why do I feel like I have not gotten back my physical stamina?

We have heard from numerous triumphers that they have not been able to get back to their before-cancer achievements in physical activities. For instance, if they were runners, they cannot run as far without feeling tired. If they were tennis players, they do not think they can play as many sets as they were once able to do. There have been a few studies in this area, showing that people were still complaining about feeling tired three to four years after treatment had ended. It's difficult, however, to separate the problems of getting older from the side effects of treatment. It's also hard to know whether these people are more aware of their bodies and looking more closely at how they react. It's important to continue physical activities, trying to build yourself up bit by bit without overexerting yourself. Most important of all, listen to your body. If you feel tired, stop what you are doing and take a rest.

Is it usual to have strong reactions on anniversary dates, dates of diagnosis, etc.?

Many people have these reactions. The first, second, fifth, and tenth years seem to cause the most anxiety. Normal life changes—weddings, having children, or starting a new job—can be difficult because they are reminders of what might not have been. For most people, however, after the initial reaction, appreciation for life and the excitement of being able to live it to the fullest takes over.

WHEN BAD THINGS HAPPEN TO GOOD PEOPLE,
THEY BECOME BETTER PEOPLE.

What is meant by recurrence?

A recurrence means that the cancer has recurred—it has happened again. It means that the disease that had been inactive, or thought to have been cured, has become active again. It means that abnormal cells have begun growing and multiplying, breaking away from the original tumor and traveling through the lymph system or bloodstream to start new growths. In recurrence, the cancer that reappears is the same type as the original cancer—no matter where in the body it appears. For example, if you previously had breast cancer and it recurs in the lung, what you are diagnosed as having is breast cancer that has spread to the lung, rather than lung cancer. Local recurrence means that the cancer has come back in the same place as the original cancer. A regional recurrence means that the problem is in an area close to the original cancer. Other recurrences are called metastases or metastatic recurrence. In this case, the cancer has spread to organs or other tissues away from the original cancer, in another part of the body.

Does worry about a recurrence ever disappear?

Fears of a recurrence generally recede as time goes by, though they may never totally disappear. The anxiety of worrying that every little ache and pain is somehow connected to your cancer diagnosis is a background feeling that most cancer triumphers can relate to. But most people with cancer are able to put these thoughts aside and get on with living their normal lives. Support groups which encourage open discussion and the perfecting of relaxation techniques can be useful in easing the tendency to anxiety.

Some people, however, are unable to put their fear of recurrence aside, anticipating problems that don't exist, never for a moment forgetting their cancer experience, allowing it to overshadow their lives. If, after a year or more, you find yourself overburdened with constant uneasiness, you should consider getting help from a psychotherapist who can enable you to resolve your underlying fears. So many long-term problems are attached to living with cancer, yet many people feel they must deal with all of them without help from others. Availing yourself of the expertise of people who have dealt with problems like yours before doesn't mean you are not coping well. It means you want to be able to cope more effectively. You owe it to yourself and to your peace of mind to unburden yourself and allow yourself to be helped.

What can I do about a fear of recurrence that just seems to have come out of nowhere?

Some people who think they have buried fears completely sometimes find them returning after a few years, more strongly than ever. If you are unable to shake these feelings and find yourself dwelling on them more and more, it may be helpful to arrange a few sessions with a social worker or a psychotherapist who can help you resolve your feelings.

How can social workers be helpful?

Many of us think of social workers as part of the welfare system and don't realize that they are an important part of the medical system—and especially helpful to those who have to deal with cancer. They act as troubleshooters and problem solvers, and can be helpful in medical, financial, emotional, religious, and employment areas. Every hospital has social workers who are especially trained to provide support and help when emotional problems crop up. Though facilities and resources vary, social workers can also help in finding support groups or other trained psychological help.

Who can help me find someone to go to?

Check with your doctor or with the hospital where you have had your treatment. The Cancer Information Service and the American Cancer Society also are good places to call for help in finding the right avenue for you. They will be able to direct you to specialized support groups that many triumphers say are their lifelines to stability. If you need to talk in a one-to-one fashion, there are numerous people who specialize in treating people with cancer.

What if I just feel like running away from it all?

Running away from worries and problems is a natural reaction after you've been through a frightening and unbearable situation. Psychologically, picking up where you left off may take longer than physical healing. Your emotional well-being is so important that you must listen to what your inner self is telling you. If this feeling persists, perhaps you should consider giving yourself the luxury of some special freedom— whether it be in the form of time away from home and family, time away from work to catch up with yourself at home, or time to do something special that you've always wanted to do. Your body is telling you it needs time to recharge. Listen to it and give yourself the psychological benefit of renewed energy.

What if I can't get away, but can't get rid of the feelings of depression?

Nothing is worse than bottling up your feelings. Of course, there are many ways to release this kind of feeling—through exercise, relaxation techniques, support groups, prayer. A number of cancer triumphers we know have used what seems like a simple method that is worth trying. Instead of fighting your feelings of self-pity, go into a quiet room where you can close the door and be alone. If that isn't possible, sit in the park or in your car by yourself in a quiet spot. Set a time limit of 10 or 15 minutes (or more if you feel you need it) and allow yourself that time to whisper—or shout, if you prefer—all the complaints you have about your fate. It's wonderful to be able to complain without being a burden to another soul. When it's all over, you will probably be amazed at how much better you'll feel.

"Remember that if your cancer returns, the newer treatments may be better and second recoveries are possible."

Modified radical mastectomy, 1987, at age 67

Is it normal for me to keep thinking about how I would handle finding out I had a recurrence?

This is something that lurks in the back of most cancer survivors' minds—and it is helpful to think about how you would manage if you discovered that cancer had recurred. Many people who have had a recurrence say that the knowledge gained from the first go-around is extremely helpful in getting proper care as quickly as possible and in sifting through the possible options. Many of the same treatment options will be available. Sometimes your own oncologist may not have access to newer drugs and treatment options. It's helpful to investigate the latest drugs, treatments, and combination therapies being offered at the Comprehensive Cancer Centers. No matter what the situation, there are always available therapies that can be tried, if you are willing to take the risks involved.

What if there is a recurrence?

Recurrences do occur, and there is usually treatment available. It is important to be informed about the possibility of recurrences for your type of cancer. It is a fact that many people who have had cancer may at some time be faced with a recurrence. Some people feel that this means that nothing they have done worked for them and that they have failed. Most people are more frightened when they find they have a recurrence than they were when they were originally diagnosed. There is often a leaden feeling of failure, of total loss of control, of shock.

It's wise to arm yourself ahead of time, to be aware of the possibilities, to understand the chronic nature of cancer, to make yourself knowledgeable about what might happen, so that you'll be somewhat prepared. However, no matter how much preparation or pre-thinking you've done, the diagnosis will again leave you in a state of confusion. But, having been there before, you know the ropes. Your past knowledge and coping strengths will help you through.

Does having a recurrence mean that there's no hope for me?

Many people make that assumption—and they couldn't be further from the truth. Don't try to make any assumptions about the meaning of the recurrence until you have had plenty of time to have all the tests that need to be run completed and analyzed. So many people, during this crisis time, assume that nothing can be done. Many people try to make critical family and personal decisions during an emotionally charged period. Postpone decisions. Families often are even more discouraged than the patient and mistakenly begin to prepare themselves mentally for a future without their loved one. This can be disastrous for everyone concerned. So, if you are faced with a recurrence, though it is difficult to do, take time to wait for a full diagnosis, don't make any rash decisions, don't make any changes in your life. Discuss the problem and take a wait-and-see attitude, which will serve you best through the initial period.

What can I do while I'm waiting for a complete diagnosis about my recurrence?

While you are waiting for your complete diagnosis, you will want to gather your forces to start investigating what is the best course for you to follow. You'll be anxious. You'll feel a sense of despair. That's perfectly natural and normal. Deal with those feelings, but don't try to project what will happen next. Give yourself the necessary time—anywhere from two to six weeks is what triumphers tell us is needed and is usually the amount of time before all testing is completed—to get accustomed to the new diagnosis and to start making plans about how you will deal with this new turn of events. Gather as much information as you can about any treatments being suggested for you. Talk to others who've been through the treatments. Don't be afraid to question your doctor. If you need more information, call the Cancer Information Service's 1-800-4-CANCER. Some people have told us they went to the medical library and picked up as much material as they could get their hands on about their type of cancer. Even if it's hard or impossible for you to understand, the medical literature can give you some insights into what new treatments are being used, who the doctors are who are involved in the treatment, what hospitals are involved in special treatments.

Though it may be intimidating to approach physicians, if you've done your homework, you may find it helpful to get in touch by telephone with some of those who are working in specific areas that relate to your case. Call them, identify yourself, explain that you are willing to pay for a telephone consultation, and explain your case and your questions. Quiz them about the possible side effects and the worst-case scenario. If you know ahead of time what you might expect, it will be easier to make decisions and to deal with the future. Don't be afraid to discuss any research you have seen—and be sure you ask difficult questions on how the treatments are being conducted and evaluated before you make any decisions. There are many uncertain areas, and you need to ask enough questions to make sure you are getting clear and comparable information.

How can I get the doctor to spend more time with me at the hospital so I can get the information I need?

Studies, including one recently completed by the Albany Medical College, have found that doctors spend about four to five minutes with the average patient during morning rounds in the hospital. Even though that does not seem like much time, if you are prepared you can get a lot of needed and valuable information. During these few moments, you will have the doctor's undivided attention. Prepare for the conversation. Make sure you have thought about the subject you wish to discuss. It might be useful to pick one topic you would like to talk about each time, writing down several questions you have about it. If it makes you more comfortable, get a tape recorder and tape the conversation. After you have tried these steps, if you still do not feel you are getting enough time, tell the doctor directly that you would like him to spend a little more time with you the next day as you have a list of questions you want answered. Or prepare the list and tell him these are the questions you need to discuss.

Who can help me decide where I can best be taken care of after being discharged from the hospital?

Many patients are not aware that most hospitals have discharge planners on staff with whom they can arrange an appointment. The job of the discharge planner is to help plan for care after the hospital stay—looking at the needs of the patient and family and making suggestions for meeting those needs. Discharge planning is usually coordinated by a social worker who may involve other health professionals, depending on the problem. Doctors, nurses, pharmacists, physical

or occupational therapists, and dieticians may all be part of
the process. They can arrange for nursing care, refer you to
agencies in the community who can assist you, help you find
a nursing home or home-care services. Federal law requires
that hospitals which participate in Medicare have a discharge
planning process for those patients who need it.

**Is there anything I can do to make my time waiting for
treatment less difficult to deal with?**

Both patients and families tell us they find treatment area
waiting rooms difficult to deal with, especially when cancer
recurs. Even when you are doing well and just come in for a
checkup, the waiting room may bring out feelings of grief,
anger, fear, and helplessness in you and your family. You
meet and get friendly with other patients and sometimes
look at your own problems in terms of their situations. When
other patients do poorly, it is difficult not to worry about your
own treatment. It might be useful to bring things with you to
keep you busy in the waiting room. A book to read, a puzzle
to work on, some needlework, letters that need answering—
all can be used to keep your attention on other things. Calling ahead to see if the doctor's appointments are on schedule
can help to lessen the time you need to spend in this atmosphere.

Why do I feel so angry with my doctor?

Most of us have expectations for our doctors that can be quite
unreasonable and impossible. Quite frankly, we expect our
doctors to cure us. When a cancer recurs, we feel that it's the
doctor's fault. We know it's irrational, but sometimes we just
can't help blaming the doctor for our illness. This anger is
rooted in our mistaken feelings about a doctor's infallibility.
These feeings are not healthy—and they can disrupt the
whole relationship with the doctor. If you find yourself in this
kind of situation, you should examine your feelings and if you

cannot come to a happy accommodation, perhaps you might want to consider changing doctors. Before you do, though, it would be wise for you to schedule an extra 15 minutes at your next appointment to talk over the problems as you see them. Just discussing it will help to dissipate some of the frustration and anger, and should make communication easier. The doctor's business is to help you—and he can't help you unless he knows what's bothering you. Clear the air. If after a few months that still doesn't help, then perhaps it's time for you to make the break and start using another physician.

Is it true that sometimes the risks and side effects of further treatment aren't worth the benefits?

The point at which this begins to be true is always debatable. Some people feel that once they've been through treatment, that is all they care to deal with. Of course, with the ever-improving outlook of medicine today, it's important not to come to this conclusion too hastily. But it is up to each patient to weigh the pros and cons, the side effects and the aftereffects, to determine what is right in each case. In this highly personal area of decision making, it is possible only to suggest some topics that should be considered. Here are some things to think about:

- Have I gotten another opinion so that I'm certain of what all my alternatives are?
- Have I been to a major cancer center for information and consultation?
- Have I checked the PDQ (information available through the 1-800-4-CANCER information service phone number) to see what investigational treatments are available for my condition?
- Am I more interested in quality or quantity of life?
- How can I exercise control over my life?
- Have I asked the doctor what benefits he expects from treatment? What side effects? What risks? What will happen if I don't have treatment? Am I ready to stop treatment altogether?

- What is it I am most afraid of? Pain? Isolation? Leaving things undone? Being unable to take care of myself? Dying?

"I've toyed with suicide a number of times. I phoned my minister just before he left for Florida and he told me that while he was away to remember I was going through a tunnel not a cavern. That did a lot to help me. Knowing how close to the brink I have been in the past keeps me alert to signs of depression. I then call a friend, visit someone who is confined to her home, buy something new, reread the Serenity Prayer."

Hysterectomy for cancer of endometrium, 1983, at age 66

Is suicide considered by people with cancer at one time or another?

It is known that many people with cancer do go through a suicidal stage during their recuperation period or when they learn of a recurrence. Most often, with time, the person begins to feel that he or she has some control over the situation. Officially, the statistics that are available for the true incidence of suicide among those with cancer are quite scarce. A Connecticut study shows that the rate of suicide of cancer patients was the same as the rate for the normal population. However, a Finnish study shows the rate to be 30 to 90 percent higher. In Sweden, about 20,000 persons a year die of cancer and only 20 to 25 of them die from suicide according to their statistics.

Should you or someone you know be contemplating such a move, it's important to be able to discuss these feelings. The taboos in our society against even thinking about suicide are so strong that the tendency is to suppress or conceal any such thoughts. But as this is something many people quite normally think about in the course of their illness, it is helpful to be able to bring these feelings into the open, since there is nothing worse than feeling alone with such burdensome thoughts. Significant in studying suicides is the fact that in about half of the cases, the actions were unexpected by those who knew them. It is felt that many suicides could be prevented if those who minister to them are attentive to their needs, feelings, and thoughts. In interviews with family members and caretakers, it was found that more than half the subjects had conveyed suicide thoughts or plans to relatives in some way. In some cases, the patient had talked of committing suicide so often that the threat had ceased to elicit a reaction. Help from a crisis center should be sought, so that the person and the family and caretakers can discuss feelings with someone who has had experience in dealing with suicide, and to bring perspective to the problems and emotions that are present.

Do's and Don'ts

DO talk about what is happening in a straightforward way. No feelings are off-limits.

DO share information and feelings with everyone in the family.

DO accept help offered by others.

DO be flexible about your demands on yourself and your family.

DO modify your standards if necessary to make life easier for everyone.

DO remember that time will help everyone get used to changing situations.

DO seek professional help if, after a reasonable amount of time, you're still struggling with problems.

DO express the love you feel to family and friends.

DO remember that you have to live only one moment at a time.

DO concentrate on recovery rather than survival.

DON'T try to tackle your whole problem at once.

DON'T make hasty decisions. Give yourself and your situation time.

DON'T be afraid.

DON'T be afraid to be happy and to enjoy what is fun, good, and beautiful.

DON'T expect too much of yourself too soon.

DON'T waste energy worrying.

DON'T give up hope.

chapter 7

For Parents of Young People with Cancer

The diagnosis of a child with a life-threatening disease is one of the greatest challenges any parent can face, laden with intense emotions, charged with anxiety, and intensified by fear. Accepting that the diagnosis is a fact is the first step in mobilizing your efforts so that you can come to grips with the reality that your child has cancer. Though the emotional pain is great, the parent's role is clearly defined, and normal parental instincts give children a strong feeling of being cared for and protected. Children are suddenly called upon to deal with adult-sized problems, and are faced with fears of pain and uncertainty. We want to wrap their thoughts in a soft, warm blanket and tell them not to worry, that we will take care of everything. Yet this is not possible. Feeling even more vulnerable than they normally do, children with cancer are faced with hospital stays and procedures that seem cruel and unfair. Yet the bravery and courage of young cancer patients is a monument to the resiliency of youth. The statistics for children with cancer, with healthy cells triumphing over cancerous ones, have improved so sharply year by year that the job is usually not one of preparing your child for death, but rather for living with a chronic illness.

Is it really wise to tell a child he or she has cancer?

"What can we say?" is one of the most difficult questions parents have to grapple with. In the past, many parents tried to shield the child from knowing. After years of experience, the consensus is that people should be told as much about the illness as their age allows them to understand. Studies have shown that even when children are not told, they grasp the meaning of what is happening, they overhear discussions, and most of them are able to understand that they are facing a life-threatening situation, made all the more frightening because no one will talk with them directly about it.

Who is the best equipped to tell the child?

A great deal depends upon the age and maturity of the child —but many parents prefer to tell the child themselves. Some prefer to have the doctor present, others prefer to discuss it with the child alone. Some parents choose to have the doctor explain. You must choose whatever way is best for you.

How can I help my child to accept what is happening?

All people who have cancer, especially children, need to be reassured that cancer is a serious but treatable disease. They need to be reassured that the cause of cancer is unknown, that treatments may be part of their lives for a long time. Many children have the impression from watching television that everyone who has cancer (especially leukemia) dies. They need to know that there are successful treatments and that new treatments are bringing hopeful results. Your attitude and the way you view their sickness will be reflected in their attitudes. If you maintain an attitude of honesty and hope, you'll see that attitude grow in them.

What feelings and fears should I be aware of so that I can reassure my child?

Guilt and anger are feelings that most children must deal with during severe illness. Guilt feelings often stem from the subconscious feeling that sickness is a punishment for having misbehaved. Very often children feel helplessly angry at themselves or at you for allowing this illness to happen. Make it possible for your child to tell you about the guilt and anger. Recognize it for what it is and remember that even a child who is angry with you loves you. You need to be able to assure children that the disease is not anyone's fault and that everyone is doing everything possible to make things better. Wrap them with love, let them know what is happening, and allow them to express fears of death openly. This is an outlet children with cancer need to have, and though it is painful to deal with, it gives you the opportunity to comfort and to reassure.

Do children who have been told they have cancer when they are first diagnosed do better psychologically than those who are told later?

A study of 116 children who had survived childhood cancer found that those who had been told about their illness earliest were in better psychological condition than those who were not told for a year or more or who discovered the truth on their own.

When should the child's brothers and sisters be told?

Though age and maturity of other children must be considered, some explanation should be given to brothers and sisters as soon after the diagnosis as possible. Children are aware of trips to the doctors, hospitalization, and other events in the household. They are frightened by the sadness they see on the faces of parents and other family members and friends. To save them from the frustration of guessing what is happening, it is best to keep them updated day by day, explaining the facts in a way that is understandable for their age and maturity. If they are very young, you may just want to say that their brother or sister is very sick, will have to stay in the hospital for a while, and will need to take medicine for a long time. Older children should be given more detailed information about cancer. As treatments are given, you will want to prepare the siblings for the physical changes, such as hair loss.

What kind of concerns do siblings have that I should be aware of?

Many children say that they worry because they have said things like "I hate you," "Drop dead," "I wish you were never born," to their brothers or sisters and feel as though they are responsible for the illness. Such feelings should be discussed and dispensed with so that they do not cause problems later on. Children also worry that cancer may be contagious and that they will be sick if they touch the patient. They need to be reassured that this will not happen, that they are healthy and that the possibility of others in the family having cancer is unlikely. Children also worry about how much the needles and blood tests and treatment hurt, and feel guilty about feeling so good themselves while their sibling is so ill. It's a good idea to encourage the other children to make cards and keep in communication with the ill child and to arrange for them to visit the hospital so they can understand what is being done when a painful procedure or strange machinery is being discussed.

Feelings of jealousy often surface during the time of treatment. Though they know it's irrational, siblings may feel upset over what they see as special privileges of the ill child

—not having to go to school, getting special gifts, being given special things to eat. Try to get them to talk about these feelings so that you can explain that they are perfectly normal. Take this opportunity to explain that you are not abandoning them by being away so much, that you love them as much or more than you always have and that you, too, hope that life will get back to normal very soon.

Is it common for siblings of cancer patients to have behavior problems?

Other children in the family often have a difficult time with the many changes in their lives that result from the disruption of a child in the family with cancer. They may become depressed, complain of illness, or begin to act out at school or in the neighborhood. If teachers are alert to the problems in the home, they can alert you when problems arise at school. Sometimes it is helpful to seek a few counseling sessions for siblings to help them sort out their feelings. The staff at the treatment center may have experience in this area and may be able to help you with this.

How should the child's classmates be told about his or her cancer condition?

This question has been grappled with by many parents and teachers. Many school districts have special programs designed to help children understand illness and disability. Some school districts require prior written permission of parents of each class member before the illness of a classmate can be discussed. Being in touch with school personnel as soon as possible and on a continuing basis is the best insurance that the child's needs will be met. When young people understand the background of a classmate's cancer and treatment, they are less likely to make ill-considered remarks. If the embarrassing side effects, such as temporary weight loss or hair loss, are explained, most young people are understanding and supportive. Classmates with questions should be encouraged to ask them.

How do you deal with classmates who tease a child about hair loss and other changes in appearance?

When the situation is explained in simple terms, most children rise to the occasion and even become defenders and champions of the child with cancer. Sometimes, however, teasing may be the result of classmates feeling that the student with cancer gets unfair attention, pampering, or special considerations beyond what is really necessary. This type of behavior can also result when a classmate is personally frightened by the situation. If your child who has cancer has problems with other children, do not hesitate to communicate with school personnel so that behavior may be modified or changed.

"Cancer forced me to grow up a lot faster than other kids my age. I tried to stay as involved with my school as I was before my illness. This helped me to stay normal. My advice to parents is to be supportive but not to 'baby' the child with cancer."

Diagnosed with non-Hodgkin's lymphoma in 1984 at age 16

Why is it important to try not to overprotect the child who is ill with cancer?

Aside from the fact that overprotection breeds an inconsiderate and demanding person, it is important in other respects as well. Overprotection encourages dependency that prevents the child from learning how to use his own resources to best meet the challenges that the disease may require. Self-confidence can also be undermined by overprotection. Be sure to discuss special activities—such as sports—with the doctor and get advice on whether they can be continued. If the doctor sees no reason to discontinue these activities, then you should not deny participation but encourage it. Of course, if medications make a child very tired, then you should be aware of this and help the child to make the decision about how much to undertake.

How much discipline should you impose on a child who has been through the cancer experience?

Discipline is important to the growth of every child—but disciplining a child who has been ill and in pain is often hard for parents. Discipline is a necessary and important life training for all children, whether or not they are ill. Even when you find it difficult because of uncertainty for the future, you need to remind yourself that setting boundaries for behavior and activity is a valuable part of growing up and doubly important for the child who may be faced with more uncertainty in the future.

What special considerations should be made for high school students with cancer?

Our experience with high school students has been that they are among the most positive of cancer patients—coping in a normal fashion with daily living and school activities. Although cancer can interfere with the adolescent's attempts to achieve independence from parents and other adults, sensitivity to possible conflicts can help to smooth the way for everyone concerned. The developmental issues facing adolescents—independence, peer acceptance, body image, and self-worth—as well as the mechanics and policies of the operation of a large school, all must be considered.

Larger classes and greater numbers of teachers may make it more difficult for the young person to maintain contact with the school during treatment periods. Such policies as rules against wearing hats in class may create embarrassment

for the student without hair when a teacher who is unaware
of the illness demands that the hat be removed. A large part
of the solution to such problems lies in good communication.
It is helpful if one person in the school can be made responsible for contact with parents and medical staff and for dissemi-
nating information to all teachers involved with the student.
Guidance counselors can be a great help in making good
communication possible.

**Is it common for teenage patients to complain about over-
protection?**

This is a common complaint of patients—as well as of teenagers everywhere—but it can pose special problems for adolescents with cancer. The disease forces them, at a time
when they are seeking independence, to be dependent upon
their parents and doctors. One of the most successful ways of
dealing with this is to allow the teenager to be involved as
much as possible in decisions that need to be made concerning medical treatment options. You can be helpful by assuring hospital personnel that they do not need to "beat around
the bush," that your child will be involved in hearing about
treatment and progress and in helping make decisions as to
what is to be done. Most young people mature during their
cancer treatments and are well able to see their way clearly
to being involved in the decision-making process.

**Is it possible for most children with cancer to continue going
to school?**

Young people with cancer can, in most instances, continue to
attend school and can benefit from attending school while
continuing their treatments. Planning and determination are
helpful in making school attendance possible. There may
have to be some absences for medical reasons, but most are
not insurmountable. You will need the cooperation of the
medical team so that treatments can be planned with the goal

of having the patient miss as little school as possible. Chemo-therapy can, for instance, be given after school hours or on weekends. It may take some doing, but it is worth discussing with your doctor. Communication with school officials and planning with school personnel can be used to good effect in making it possible for almost every child with cancer to ben-efit from the educational and social advantages of the school experience.

Does a child with cancer have special rights under the law?

Public Law 94-142, passed by the U.S. Congress and signed into law by President Gerald Ford in November 1975, re-quires that every state provide a free and appropriate educa-tion in the least restrictive environment for all handicapped individuals between the ages of 3 and 21. Therefore, the public school is mandated by the federal government through PL 94-142 to provide an appropriate education for students with cancer whose medical problems adversely af-fect their educational performance. Continuation of schooling gives the child hope and should be the goal as soon as the child is medically able. If it seems like your child will have to miss school for any length of time, it is wise to ask for an assessment and consideration of Special Education place-ment as soon after diagnosis as possible. This should be done through the clinic or hospital by one of the professionals—doctor, nurse, social worker, psychologist, hospital teacher, or school liaison person. An assessment will be made through testing, and an Individual Education Plan, which you will hear referred to as an IEP, is then prepared. It will be de-signed to provide the student with the class placement and services most appropriate to fit the needs. One person is usually designated to become the liaison with the hospital or clinic team and to coordinate activities. Some of the services that are available include:

- Special tutoring for subjects in which the child has fallen behind because of frequent treatments or illness-related absences.

- Instruction at home or in the hospital when the child must be out for more than a few days.
- Specialized physical education if needed.
- Special arrangements for taking makeup tests.
- Waiver of automatic absence penalties.
- Assistance of school nurse or other health office personnel in administering drugs.
- Liaison with regular class teachers to inform them of special needs.

What kind of information do I have to provide to school personnel so that my child can continue going to school?

If the teaching team is fully informed about the student's treatment, your child should be able to continue as normal a school routine as possible. Some of the information that should be shared includes:

- An explanation of the specific type of cancer and how it is being treated.
- What kind of treatment is being given, how and when it is administered, what the side effects may be, and what effects there are on behavior and appearance.
- The approximate schedule of upcoming treatment, procedures, or tests that may result in the student's absence.
- Some information on how the student is reacting to the illness, how informed the student is about the illness and treatment.
- What limitations, if any, the health-care team has placed on the student's activities.
- Whether the student prefers to discuss the illness with teachers and/or other students.
- How the student's siblings are dealing with the problem.

Is it wise to get the student's doctor, nurse, and/or social worker together with teachers, parents, and student to work out solutions to school situations?

Sometimes this is the most direct way to handle a difficult school situation. If the treatment center is close, it is possible to make arrangements for a conference so that a joint plan can be drawn up. Even if it is not possible to involve all parties, it is helpful to put together a consistent plan. Appointing one teacher, counselor, administrator, or school nurse as the liaison between the school, the family, and the treatment center has been one approach that works well. The person chosen should be willing to assume responsibility for keeping teachers of the patient as well as teachers of siblings informed.

How do you keep from overprotecting a child with cancer in the classroom?

Finding a balance is a daily problem—and one that will need to be assessed regularly, because cancer cannot be ignored, but neither can other important aspects of the young person's life. The same limits on behavior should apply to students with cancer as to their classmates. Special treatment in the classroom can create resentment among peers. Although the diagnosis of cancer will change your child's life for a time, the same needs remain as other young people—for friends, school, and activities. Friendships can be kept alive through letters and telephone calls, if the child is being hospitalized. You should encourage your child to continue to live as normally as possible during this time.

What kinds of problems do parents themselves face while their children are undergoing treatment?

Parents become great advocates for their children. They learn everything there is to be known about the disease, what the treatments are, when they need to be given, and what side effects they produce. They usually carry this information with them when the children go to the hospital for their treatments and many times they know as much as the doctor does about their child's illness. They usually give selflessly of themselves. Many parents tell us that their moods during the treatment period depend upon what is happening. When the treatments are going well, the parents' moods are high. When there are problems, their moods reflect them. It may be hard for parents to separate themselves from their child's illness. Some say they even feel guilty going out with their friends. Be prepared for the many mood swings and for feeling that you've been dealt a difficult hand. Make sure you take some time for yourself. This is not the time to be a martyr. Rather, it's a time to make special efforts to be kind to yourself and your partner. You both need to get away from the rigors of dealing with a sick child every once in a while.

What special summer arrangements are there for children with cancer?

The American Cancer Society and other groups such as children's hospitals, civic groups, and the Ronald McDonald Houses support camping programs for children with cancer. There are approximately 100 such programs around the country. The programs, the locations, and the activities vary from wilderness camping to day camps. Boating, fishing, swimming, relay races, art classes are all part of the fun. At most camps, health professionals, doctors, nurses, and social workers donate their vacations to be part of the camp team.

There are camps in just about every state. Some are only for children with cancer; others allow brothers and sisters to come. Some include children with other chronic diseases; most allow children who are taking oral chemotherapy to participate. All have medical staffs. Many of the camps, especially those run by the American Cancer Society, are free to state residents. At others, the costs range from $20 to $300 for sessions lasting from two days to two weeks. Some scholarships are available. For more information on camps in your area, see Chapter 9, or call the local office of the American Cancer Society or any major medical center that treats children with cancer.

What kinds of problems do children and adolescents with cancer face even when their future is a physically healthy one?

Unfortunately, there is a certain amount of discrimination against individuals cured of cancer. For example, survivors of childhood cancer are currently not eligible for any type of military service, regardless of their health status. Insurance is also a problem, since some civilian employers feel that the cancer could recur at any time. Candlelighters' (a national group for parents with children who have cancer) parent support groups are leading a campaign to change these ingrained attitudes. Even some school systems make it difficult for cancer patients to have their individual educational needs met. However, Public Law 94-142 (as previously explained) mandates that every school provide an appropriate education for cancer patients whose medical problems adversely affect their school performance.

Do children sometimes encounter other health problems after being successfully treated for cancer?

There have been a number of studies done to determine some of the issues that are involved with children who survive cancer now that more children are surviving for longer periods of time, and thus are more likely to develop late complications of aggressive therapies. A variety of learning problems have been noted in some children following treatment. Certain types of radiation of the cranial areas and some chemotherapy may cause impairment of perception and motor function as well as intellectual capacity. Some children who receive chemotherapy may lose part of the sensation in their fingers, making it difficult for them to write well; others report that they are more easily distracted, a result of disrupted roles and emotional upsets. Other issues include possible genetic implications, sterility, dental problems, and fear of second malignancies. Irradiation in the brain area may include the pituitary gland and can have an effect on reducing the amount of growth hormone produced so that the treated child fails to grow to his full height.

Cancer treatments can themselves sometimes lead to cancer—so it is important to remember that children cured of cancer must be followed closely by their physicians for life, not only to ensure that the original cancer remains under control, but to detect the development of any late complications which may require corrective measures. These problems did not exist even a few years ago, because for so many children with cancer there was no hope. As more and more of these children become adults, more is being learned about how best to deal with these late aftereffects.

Do children with cancer end up having more emotional problems than others?

Most young people adjust quite well to having cancer, with little long-term damage to self-esteem. A recent study shows that it's wise to educate adolescents with cancer. The study showed that the more patients understand about their disease, the higher their self-image.

What groups are available to help parents and children cope with cancer?

One group that is expressly designed for parents and children who are coping with cancer is Candlelighters, founded in 1970. It is the oldest and largest of the pediatric networking organizations and has established links with 250 cancer support groups nationally and internationally. In addition to self-help groups which encourage support for the sick child and his or her parents and family, the group publishes newsletters, distributes handbooks, operates a telephone hotline, is developing training materials for long-term survivor and youth leadership groups, and is involved in advocacy issues like special education, medical leave policies, employment, and insurance. Information is available by writing: Candlelighters Foundation, 1901 Pennsylvania Avenue, NW, Suite 1001, Washington, DC 20006; telephone: 202-659-5136. (See Chapter 9 for more information.)

chapter 8

For Family and Friends

It's not easy being on the other side of the bed, hearing the news that someone you love has cancer. Many people have the idea that because a person has cancer, he or she is going to die. Some people do die from cancer. But many people live for a long time with the illness. Increasing numbers of people are surviving cancer. Five million living Americans have been treated. Of the Americans diagnosed with cancer today, more than half will live a normal life span. If you hold on to the outdated thinking that there's no hope for people with cancer, you'll make it very hard for the person you love who has it—and you'll make it very hard for yourself as well. So, the first lesson to be learned is: DON'T MAKE ANY ASSUMPTIONS. Don't panic. Try not to carry on in a hysterical fashion.

There are many, many factors that need attention during the beginning stages, and family and friends must rally together to make it possible for the patient to use energy to rally his or her own forces in the most positive way possible to face what's ahead. Try to keep life as normal as possible in spite of a situation that is going to require everyone to make some changes.

Expect to feel confused and fearful, angry, guilty, and sad. Expect to go through feelings that are related to those you feel when you mourn someone's death. Expect to hear those same sentiments echoed by the family member who has cancer. Listen for the anger, the guilt, the questioning of God, and other emotions that are part of the mourning process.

How do you respond? Affirm that it is a terrible blow. But also affirm hope. Since each person is different, reactions will vary, so listen carefully. Many people who have received a cancer diagnosis say that they are so wrapped up in their own chaotic world of shock that they find it hard to communicate. Being honest about your own feelings and fears, and encouraging the same honesty from the patient, will lift the burden of putting up a front. Facing up to reality won't make the problems go away, but it will make them easier to cope with.

Don't be afraid to cry with your family member or good friend. We all need to talk about our fears—and we need to talk about them with those who care about us the most, not with acquaintances or business colleagues, but with those who are nearest to us. Yet triumphers tell us that, often, that's the hardest thing to do. Many people find it most difficult to reveal their innermost anxieties to those they love because they want to protect them from their panic. That kind of protection can only result in tensions building up on both sides and new barriers being formed. If you can start off with honest communication, you've made the most important step in moving forward and dealing with the reality of cancer.

Is it usual for the family as well as the patient to go into a state of shock at first?

Accepting a diagnosis of cancer, with all the fear it carries with it, usually pushes the patient and everyone around him into a state of shock and denial. Even more difficult to deal with is the state of confusion that follows, while the diagnosis is being confirmed and tests are being done to determine what will be the best course of treatment to follow. All of this testing and planning takes a great deal of time, with the patient and family left "hanging" in an atmosphere of confusion. To help combat these feelings, you may want to turn your attention to gathering information on the specific kind of cancer, combing the medical literature, talking with specialists, and working to get together as much material as you can so that you can help the patient to make as informed a decision as possible.

Checklist for the Family

Are you pressuring the patient to:
Stop talking about his health because it's morbid?
Stop feeling sorry for himself?
Prove that he's feeling great even when he isn't?

Instead, help by:
Letting him talk about his problems and finding positives to talk about.
Keeping his interest up about home, work, and world affairs.
Being sympathetic but emphasizing the good things about life.
Not pressuring him to be a cheerleader to *you* to keep up *your* spirits.
Letting him level with you about his feelings.

What can I say to a friend who I've just learned has cancer?

Saying the right thing isn't a matter of coming up with a pat phrase that covers every occasion. Being frightened by the image that someone we love is dying often leaves us silent, with a void that can be misinterpreted by the patient. Jory Graham, whose column, "A Time for Living," was syndicated in 50 newspapers, during the time she had cancer said that the most remarkable statement ever made to her by a friend upon hearing her news was "Jory, that's a tragedy." Another friend simply said, "Oh, Jory," but reached for her hand, and a third said, "Care to tell me more?" Some, she reported, simply had tears in their eyes. It isn't always what we say, but how we react. Even if you've always been reserved, express your caring with a hug. Most importantly, don't try to hide your feelings and turn away. Don't stop calling or visiting because you feel uncomfortable. If you feel uncomfortable, say so.

How can you deal with a cancer patient who is hopeless and depressed and wants to give up?

Feelings of depression are a part of accepting the cancer diagnosis. This kind of hopelessness and depression often strikes cancer patients—and sometimes a quest for information helps to pull them out of the dumps. You might feel tempted to go along with the depression because of your own deep-down feelings that cancer is a hopeless disease. But you won't be helping the patient or yourself by doing that. Being passive only lays the groundwork for future problems. Sometimes acknowledging the sadness by saying something like "You don't complain, but it must be terrible" may help to start the conversation so that worries and anger can be expressed. Moving forward by trying to instigate an interest in the need to make decisions can also be helpful. What is the best treatment to choose? Is this doctor the best one? What new treatments are being talked about? Where are they being done? Avoid being falsely cheerful or optimistic. Instead, try to deal with the true facts of the situation and help make plans for how to deal with the reality of what is happening.

"What can friends do? Just be there. It is okay to say you are scared too and you do not know what to say or do. Nobody does. Crying with the person is fine. Just be with the person as much as you can."

Diagnosed with inoperable lung cancer in 1984 at age 46, now in remission after radiation and chemotherapy treatment

---

Why am I so afraid to face the fact that my own biggest fear is of death?

Regardless of how good the prognosis is, none of us can help but think about death when faced with a life-threatening disease such as cancer. In our society, where everyone tries to ignore dying, and can, because the reality of dying is not something that is part of our everyday lives, a cancer diagnosis forces us to look at the unknown. Most families admit that this is one of their biggest, most unresolved fears. Again, if it is at all possible, try to discuss your fears along with your hopes for the future. Admit that you're frightened. Let people know how important they are to your life. Realize that today, many patients have a normal life span, but for those whose life may be shortened by cancer, it is a disease that gives a transition time between life and death, conveying to everyone concerned time to learn to prepare for what is inevitable eventually for us all.

Why do I feel so angry at my family member who has cancer?

Like the feelings of shock and fear, anger is another emotion that surfaces and often takes us by surprise. Whatever the patient's role, it is an important one in the family, and the family will feel angry that the role is being disrupted. "How will we manage without you?" is the family's battle cry. This may bring about one of two reactions—pushing or pulling. The family may react by telling the patient he must get well and swing into action by trying to push him into getting better. Other families react in just the opposite fashion—by pulling away. The unconscious act is the result of being so threatened by the fear of death that they back away to spare themselves from hurt. People who react in this way try to run away from their feelings by withdrawing into their work or other outside activities that keep them from the ill member of the family. However, if you can understand this feeling of anger, the family can learn to cope with it and deal with it in a more positive way, by expressing love and affection for each other and bringing about a closer bonding of the family group.

How can adolescents be helped to cope with a parent's cancer?

It has been discovered that adolescents often find it comforting to learn all about their parent's disease and to participate closely with the health-care team. They can be encouraged to use information gathering as a way of gaining a certain sense of control over a difficult-to-understand situation. Beyond that, many adolescents are able to develop philosophic depth that helps them to grasp the meaning and value of their relationship with their parents. Sometimes when a parent is very seriously ill, the problems of adolescence seem to become acute. Problems at school and with siblings and family are often the teenager's way of trying to force someone to pay attention. This is an unconscious way of letting parents know how much they are needed. The usual course of adolescence, where the teenager undergoes the normal process of devaluing parents and their values, may be impeded—when a parent has a serious illness—by feelings of guilt and fear. Sometimes, this results in overidealizing the ill parent and directing hostility toward the well parent. Understanding the possibility of these patterns of behavior can be helpful in enabling teenagers and families alike to deal with their feelings.

Why is it that the whole family seems to be affected by the fact that one member has cancer?

The observation has been made that cancer is a family disease because it does affect the whole family. To avoid negative and detrimental attitudes, it is important for the family to realize that their own adjustments to cancer are as crucial as the patient's adjustment. Everyone in the family will have fears, negative attitudes, and insecurities that need to be addressed. Being able to say, "I'm scared," and to get beyond the empty talk, empty anger, and falseness is what the whole family needs. When death threatens one person in the family (whether or not it is due to occur now or at a distant time is unimportant), it threatens all. We have a taboo in our culture that makes it hard to talk about death. But talking about the possibility of death and our feelings about it is the first step in coming to grips with the problem and an important part of recovery.

Should we tell the patient and other people about the cancer diagnosis?

This is the hardest question for many people—and one that has to be faced squarely at the very start. It was a more difficult question in the days when cancer was inevitably fatal. But even in those days, the truth was less painful than denial. Today, when there are many treatments, choices, and options, and so much hope for recovery, it is imperative that honesty be used in dealing with the question. Dying is part of the experience of living. Avoiding the discussion puts a distance between the patient and the rest of the world that becomes impossible to bridge. By denying the truth, all parties have a harder time. The patient becomes isolated. The family is stranded with their denial. Friends are locked out. No one is allowed to express his true feelings. Anger is suppressed. True expression is blocked. This gives alarming signs of fear to the patient—far more damaging than facing the truth. Your initial reaction may be to protect the patient from facts that you feel the person cannot face. Experience has shown that in almost every case, the patient knows anyway. Advice from every quarter is: do not try to keep the diagnosis a secret.

What happens in cases when the diagnosis or prognosis of cancer isn't discussed with the patient or is denied by the patient?

Experience has shown that first of all, most people, whether they are told or not, instinctively know when they have cancer. This forces the patient, the family, and the health-care team to live with the lie, continuing to conceal true feelings and emotions. The reaction snowballs into further denial, distrust, avoidance of reality, and isolation. Many times, the emotional burden evolves into depression. No two people react in exactly the same way since everyone has different emotions, fears, and concerns, but honest discussion of the diagnosis and prognosis has been shown to allow the patient to most comfortably make whatever adjustments are necessary in the least stressful environment.

Why do I find myself worrying so much about my future when my spouse is the one with the cancer diagnosis?

It's not unusual to be overwhelmed with a jumble of feelings —and to feel guilty because you cannot be totally sensitive to your partner's emotions because you are concerned about what will happen to you in the future. You are going through exactly the same menu of feelings as the cancer patient— only in terms that pertain to you, which is perfectly normal. All of us feel anger and self-pity at having to deal with unwanted illnesses. The important thing to remember is that you need to adopt a positive attitude to help you in coping— but this can take time.

Why does the patient seem to be pushing me out of his life, treating me no more personally than he does his nurse?

It has been observed that, during times of stress, some patients reject those closest to them, those they love the most. The reasons are complicated and psychological—but they have to do with the patient's guilt at putting you through this difficult time. When understood in that context, it is easier to deal with the feelings of rejection that come over you and will help in guiding you to find the right words to help break down this rejection.

What should a family do to be most helpful to the patient?

During the first few weeks, while going through the period of shock that everyone feels, you can be helpful by being available, being supportive, and gathering information. One of the most important phone calls you can make is to 1-800-4-CANCER, the phone number for the Cancer Information Service, which is available across the United States to answer questions about cancer. Booklets and the latest information about every kind of cancer are available with a simple telephone call. Names of hospitals and specialists can be suggested. A computerized search for the latest investigational treatments can be made. Trained staff will answer your questions—and send you information. This is a free service that is available to everyone. Take advantage of it.

Talking with doctors, being available to participate in hospital conferences, acting as cheerleaders for the patient are all important roles for the family. The most important aspect of family involvement is being ther∙ with the patient to give as much support as possible and as much positive feedback as is appropriate. You must realize that the patient is very involved with himself at this time, so will have little time and energy left to think about others. This can leave the family feeling neglected and empty. Often the family refuses to discuss these feelings or even to face the fact that they exist. Then unhappiness builds up to major proportions and explodes in anger and depression.

The well-meaning family often feels that the patient has so many problems to cope with that they don't want to burden him with theirs. This, in effect, isolates the patient from everyday living and, in the long run, will separate the family even further. It's important to keep the lines of communication open and honest to avoid such separation. If necessary, reach out to your minister, doctor, social worker, therapist, family counselor, or good friends to air and clarify your fears, thoughts, and concerns.

"Friends and family who made 'you'll make it' remarks and offered love and prayers along the way keep you going. I've always looked ahead and kept busy at new things. I help others and see so many so much worse off than I am."

Diagnosed with breast cancer in 1979 at age 55, recurrences in 1983, 1985, and 1987

Why is the patient focusing anger on the doctor?

It has been observed, and research has confirmed, that very often in the course of an illness there needs to be someone on whom anger can be focused. Fighting the doctor, the hospital, or other members of the staff is a way of releasing all the negative feelings of anger and rage at the illness. Some doctors and nurses seem to contribute to these feelings unwittingly by appearing to be insensitive, unresponsive, or uncommunicative. Often, during the course of treatment, these feelings change and shift and many times can result in deep respect.

What if we feel it's a good idea to change doctors?

The patient should feel perfectly comfortable in seeking another opinion on his diagnosis or handling of his case. Plans will need to be discussed with your current doctor, since he will need to release medical records. Most doctors are very helpful in aiding you to seek a second opinion and may also help with referrals. Don't be afraid to help the patient take charge of the case.

When you're fighting cancer you need a doctor who considers you part of the team, and if there is a feeling of lack of trust, then change may be needed. Such change may be necessary if the doctor is not comfortable in answering questions adequately and giving you information.

But any decision to switch physicians should be based on facts, not on the hope that you'll find someone who will guarantee a cure.

What can friends do or say to be helpful?

It's often hard to know just how to behave when someone you care about has cancer and you're fearful for the future. The best thing to remember is to be as hopeful as possible, yet as honest as possible. There's a delicate balance in being hopeful because often your optimism at some points in treatment can ring untrue, giving a false message to the person who is going through the illness. Better to voice your concerns and fears and ask questions that let the patient share his thoughts with you. Touching is important—hugs, pats, handholding, kisses, and loving caresses say more than words can.

> *"Others should remember to treat cancer
> patients just as before. They're still the same
> people. Hear what they say. Listen. Don't be
> afraid to talk about cancer."*
>
> *Woman   diagnosed   with   leukemia   in   1986
> at age 46*

What are some tips on how to listen actively and give good honest advice?

There are verbal behaviors you can use that can be helpful in allowing your friends to come to grips with feelings:

- Repeat what your friend says, using slightly different words, perhaps emphasizing what you see as an important part of the message.
- Ask questions. Clarify details. This will help your friend direct attention to some of his/her as yet unconsidered issues.
- Summarize what is said and gain perspective on how it all fits together.
- Try to sort out the underlying feelings. Sometimes you'll find your friend talking around the subject he really wants to discuss.
- Indicate that what is being said makes sense to you, given what you see as the underlying feelings.
- If there's an inconsistency between what is being said and how your friend is acting, help your friend to come to grips with those feelings.

We all use certain cues to let people know we are listening and what we are thinking. These include eye signals, such as widening our eyes in disbelief, nodding our heads in agreement, murmuring our "uh, huhs" of assent. Be aware of what your responses are saying and help the other person share feelings as fully as possible.

Is it all right for me to give advice to my friend with cancer?

Advice must be given sparingly and with great care. Insensitive advice is often rejected out of hand. You have to be certain that your friend is ready and willing to accept it. The fact that someone discloses a problem does not necessarily mean she is actively looking for advice. Often, you'll find, she is just unburdening herself and needs someone to listen. One person's experience with a problem often has no relationship to someone else's problem. The more complicated the problem, the more likely it is that if a simple suggestion was really the answer, it would have already been discovered. Offering suggestions about miracle cures that have been published in the press can be the most disconcerting for patients who are dealing with the real world of their cancer. You can usually be most helpful by letting your friend talk out the problem. This frequently helps a person sort out the choices and make a decision.

How can the family help friends to be helpful?

We've all heard the offer and made it ourselves: "Just let me know what I can do to help." When we make or receive such an offer, we are sincere about wanting to help, and we need guidance in what to do. Families can help themselves as they help their friends by taking advantage of offers of assistance. Most people truly want to help, but don't want to interfere by imposing themselves on your life. Try to have a list of needs at hand and accept the help that is offered. A specific chore or errand, no matter how simple, lets your friends feel useful and makes them a part of your life. Most people are happy if there is something positive they can do to help. Think of it as a way of reaching out to others and bringing them into your family circle.

"People can help by showing love, caring, and consideration sincerely. It was helpful to have people just pitch in without having to ask."

Ovarian cancer, stage II, 1979, at age 29

What is the most practical way for the family to take advantage of friends' offers of help?

It isn't always easy to accept offers of help, either from relatives or friends. But when you are in a crisis situation, it is useful to be able to mobilize the help that is offered. People truly want to be helpful and feel better if they are given specific things to do. Make a list of tasks that others can help with—mowing the lawn, picking up the dry cleaning, shopping for groceries, taking children to lessons or after-school arrangements, providing transportation for treatments, walking the dog. We know a single woman whose friends worked out a specific schedule of needs, day by day, and sent it around to friends and acquaintances who had offered to help. There were many people who wanted to join in, and listing specific assignments allowed everyone to choose what they could do within their own schedules to help her out. Other people have handled the same kind of arrangement by sending letters to all those who had expressed an interest in helping out, allowing them to choose items from the list that they could incorporate into their own routines.

What can a family do if they just can't talk about their cancer fears?

In families where everyone feels pain but is too afraid to talk about it, it is sometimes helpful to seek a social worker, a member of the clergy, a family doctor, psychologist, or psychiatrist to help you all learn to share these difficult emotions. There are also many good programs sponsored by the American Cancer Society that use group discussions to allow professionals, people with cancer, and their families to have frank talks about their shared problems.

Is it wise for me to encourage the patient to talk about fears of dying?

Patients tell us that fears of dying come at various times during their cancer illnesses. Very early in recovery, however, every patient experiences the depression that comes from the fear of dying. There is the inevitable mourning for the loss of the feeling of stability that comes from being in good health. It is wise to encourage these feelings to be expressed —but the person with cancer is the one who must lead the way. It is important for the cancer patient to know that his fears are shared and that his feelings are understood. Don't brush off the expression of fear by assuring the patient that everything is going to be fine. That approach only makes the fear seem unimportant and encourages further denial and hopelessness. Acknowledging that death is a possibility but that you're going to do everything you can to help him recover and live offers the kind of positive comfort every patient needs. Thoughts of death occur in almost every patient; if it is at all possible, someone close to the patient should be alert to the need to talk about this, to help him to cope and to see the new meaning the cancer experience can give to his life.

How do I deal with someone who is very depressed about being sick?

Always being cheerful and optimistic in front of a patient creates an atmosphere that isn't normal—and convinces him that he's all alone with his feelings. It's better to try to be empathetic by saying, "I'm sorry you're feeling that way but I certainly understand that being so sick is depressing." By acknowledging and accepting feelings you can offer help in a way that makes the depressed person feel in control. "Is there anything I can do?" and "I'm available to help" leave openings for further discussion. Expressing your own feelings, talking about what is happening in your own life, sharing your thoughts about what is happening outside the sickbed setting also can help the patient turn attention to other things.

How do I deal with the fact that I'm the target of the cancer patient's anger and frustration?

It isn't easy. You can tell yourself that you're not the cause of the hostility—but when angry exchanges are made, it's hard not to return anger with anger. If at all possible, try to respond with compassion and understanding. Realize that even when you can't handle the situation as you might like, honest exchanges are valuable if you are able to share feelings.

What's the hardest adjustment for children of a parent who is ill with cancer?

The hardest adjustment is accepting changes in the family routine. Each age group has special problems and anxieties. Children's reactions can change from concern to frustration and resentment against the problems caused by the parent's illness. The focus of the family switches from the child to the parent. The well parent, along with all his other obligations, must take time to help the child understand. The child must be told that he plays an important role in his parent's recovery. Irritability and unreasonable behavior by the sick parent can be dealt with with maturity if the well parent has helped the youngster to come to grips with the realities of the illness. One of the most difficult reactions to deal with is the silent rejection of the stricken parent by his or her child. Although children may not discuss it, they may show rejection by ignoring advice or dealing only with the well parent. Most helpful to children in these circumstances is a well-informed listener outside the family circle who can help deal with fears and resentments.

"If you want to help, say, 'I love you,' and, 'What can I do to help?' Neighbors brought dinner to my husband and kids for six weeks. That was such a relief, knowing my family would have a nice dinner. My relatives came for a week or two in succession—one after another, nursing me and cooking batches of food to freeze for my family's later use. Getting cards from friends when I was too sick to receive visitors or phone calls was a comfort."

Diagnosed with lymphoma in 1984 at age 38

What should children be told about a cancer illness in the family?

The amount of information and the way it is presented to the child depend upon the age and intellectual maturity of the child. As a rule, a gentle, open, and honest approach is the best. Children often think that they might have caused the illness by something they did or thought. They need reassurance that nothing they did or did not do caused the illness. It is important not to try to hide what is happening from a child. Try to explain as clearly as you can what the medical procedures are, and what the disease is.

What kinds of fears do children have about the illness of a family member?

Children are afraid of death, of being abandoned by the adults around them. They fear the unknown. They recognize that there is sadness and pain around them and they do not understand the reasons for these emotions. Many children fear that information is being withheld from them—and they may suffer the same menu of feelings that adults are experiencing: anger, guilt, helplessness. It's important to include children in what is happening, sharing tears as well as joys. Let them know that you want to hear their concerns and answer their questions. Better to tell them, "No one knows for sure," than to say, "Everything will be just fine." The first is more honest and sharing; the second may tend to sound like false security.

How can young children be kept in contact with a parent who is hospitalized with cancer?

Since many hospitals will not allow young children to visit on a regular basis, the best answer is through the telephone and mail. Giving children the telephone number, and assuring them that they can call at any time, is a very reassuring gesture for those who are left behind while the parent is undergoing care. Writing letters and postcards, arranging small surprises for the children, lets them know they haven't been forgotten.

What can be done when the cancer patient becomes self-centered?

Many families complain—and feel guilty because they do— that the cancer patient becomes very self-centered and demanding. One of the most important contributions a family can make toward the recovery process is to help the patient keep his or her needs and changed living pattern in perspective with the needs of the rest of the family. Isolating the patient, catering only to his schedule, removes one whole aspect of a patient's life—the sharing, helping, giving side. This only succeeds in focusing the patient's thinking on his problems, removing him from daily life and the need to feel useful. Furthermore, it shines attention on the negative aspects of his illness, rather than on the positive aspects that are such an integral part of recovery.

- Let the patient know that how the family and the patient interact has an effect on everyone's lives.

- Strive for an honest relationship that encourages full expression and venting of emotions as well as adverse feelings, but emphasizes the positive.
- Don't be embarrassed to seek guidance from professionals, if needed. If everyone concerned does not agree to getting advice, by all means get help for yourself if you feel you need it.

Is it helpful to be falsely cheerful?

Patients tell us that there is nothing more disconcerting than false cheerfulness, and the need for some people to feel they must cheerlead the patient. This only succeeds in cutting off the patient's ability to express his true feelings. By denying reality, you force the person to withdraw because he feels you don't understand his feelings. It's better if you share your own fears and anxiety about the future.

What if I do everything for the patient and there is still no response?

Sometimes doing everything for patients is what is causing them to withdraw. People with cancer are still able to participate in their normal activities and responsibilities. Doing everything for them leaves them feeling helpless. Be very careful not to take away their decision-making opportunities. Try to let the physician know that decisions rest with the patient, not with the relatives. The whole family should be alert to the need to preserve the dignity of the patient from the feelings of dependency that can occur all too easily in the patient setting.

What if I can't give my friend who has cancer the emotional support I'd like because of my own fears?

Many people find it hard to deal with the actual fact that a friend has cancer. And, cancer patients are hurt when good friends fail to rally to their aid. They are left feeling that their friends are being disloyal when they need help most. The best way to deal with this is to talk with your friend honestly about your fears—whether they come from the fact that you've lost someone close to you through cancer and feel that you cannot invest your emotions again with someone with the same problem, or for whatever other reasons, your friend deserves an explanation.

Is it usual to lose friends as a result of having cancer?

Triumphers tell us that along the way, friends and even family members often cause disappointment. Some are confused and frightened, some just stay away, some are angry, and many change in the way they react. People rally at different times during the cancer experience. New friends appear. Many good old friends become better friends. Some people may not be at a level in their lives where they are prepared to handle this kind of crisis. As a friend, try to treat the patient as you did before. Don't act as though life is at a standstill because of cancer. Your friend hasn't changed. Only your perception of the person as a patient has changed.

What happens when the illness is prolonged and I feel I can no longer devote so much time to my friend?

Since most cancer treatments can continue for a long time, it is natural to lose that feeling of urgency to be there that you had when you first learned of the illness. It's important to understand that cancer is often a chronic illness that will continue for many years, and you cannot be expected to give the same kind of continuing attention that you did at the beginning. It is possible, also, that the patient and family are ready to look for outside support in other areas. You can start to gradually reduce your time spent with the patient, offering to do something on a routine basis, once each week or once every several weeks, so that your friend will know you continue to care.

Is it wrong for me to feel that if my partner can't be completely well, I'd prefer that he die?

This is a fairly common reaction that often changes with time. At first it sounds cruel and harsh, but understanding the psychology behind the comment makes it easier for you to deal with your own feelings. You are so strongly wishing that your spouse's pain and discomfort would disappear, that he might be spared from the ups and downs and difficulties of treatment, that you are wishing the easiest possible course for him. This is a natural reaction of someone who loves another very much, who is willing to give up that person to spare him from pain. Knowing you feel this way may be very hurtful for your spouse, though openness may allow you to feel comfortable in making such a statement directly. Be sure your partner understands the context in which you express such feelings and does not misunderstand what you are trying to say by interpreting such feelings as abandonment on your part.

How can we keep our social activities from being disrupted because of cancer treatment?

It can take the skills of a social director to keep the level of social activities going while one is combating cancer. Some friends may cease coming, relationships change, and the patient must focus attention on the problems and is unable, in some cases, to provide the necessary attention and emotional support for friends. Many relationships can be salvaged, however, if the lines of communication are kept open. At first you may want to encourage visitors to make their visits short. Tea or cocktail time is a good time for visitors. Always be sure to discuss plans with the patient so that his wishes are followed, since attempts to socialize can place a great deal of stress on a patient. It is more stressful to plan visits outside the home than it is to entertain at home at the beginning. Some families become angry when, after all the plans for an outing have been made, the patient decides not to partici-pate. When this occurs, if the patient can be left alone, per-haps the others in the family can continue with their plans. The whole family needs as much support and assurance as possible. All too often, the major consideration is focused on the patient. Directing attention to the rest of the family helps to anticipate problems and find workable solutions.

Why do I sometimes feel I must get away from the patient and all the problems of cancer and then end up feeling guilty about this?

The day-to-day business of dealing with a family member with cancer and some of its treatments over a long period is often harder on the family than on the patient. There are bound to be times when tempers are short. Then you feel the need to escape and end up feeling guilty about those feelings. In fairness to yourself and to the patient, the family should try to arrange schedules so that the responsibility is not left on the shoulders of one person only. People should be welcomed into the home and daily or weekly breaks from routine should be planned. The patient should be encour-aged to try to maintain as normal a life as is possible—con-tinuing with interests, hobbies, and social contacts. Attention should be focused away from worries about cancer.

Is it unusual that even though my partner is recovered, we still have not resumed our sexual relationship?

Chapter 4 of this book deals with some of the sexual problems that cancer patients face, and it will be helpful for you to reread this chapter so that you will have a greater understanding of some of the ramifications of cancer treatment as they relate to sex. Most cancer patients regain their sex drive as they progress in their recovery, but lack of sexual drive is not unusual and should not be viewed as a personal rejection but rather as a result of physical and emotional reaction to the illness. Many cancer patients say they experience problems in emotional concentration because of their all-encompassing concern and focus on personal health and the aftereffects of surgery and treatment. It is important for you, as the partner, to understand how deeply an illness like cancer affects the entire sense of self. The patient needs reassurance that he is loved and wanted as much as before his illness. There will be a period of adjustment and new patterns may have to be tried and learned. It may take many months before you are able to resume your sexual life as it once was. Some couples find that counseling can be helpful. Understanding and patience, and again, good communication between you, should make it possible for you to resume your sexual relationship, perhaps on a different level than before, but in a way that will be satisfying to you both.

Is it normal for me to be thinking about sex when my partner has such a serious illness?

It's perfectly natural and understandable for you to be thinking about sex even though your partner is ill. Serious illness may directly change your partner's sexuality, but the illness does not erase your own sexual needs. Hospitalization and illness may make it very difficult to spend time alone together. You need to seek ways for you and your partner to express yourselves so that your varying needs, preferences, and desires are met. Talk together about ways of maintaining sexual intimacy even if sexual intercourse is not possible. Don't hesitate to ask the doctor when sexual intercourse can be resumed.

Is it reasonable for me to have come to the conclusion that my partner is so ill and in such pain most of the time that sexual intercourse is just not a possibility for us anymore?

This is a decision that you should not make alone. You need to have a discussion with your partner and the doctor. If the outlook is that sexual intercourse is no longer possible, then it is important for you and your partner to talk about using touch and words to continue your loving relationship. Some people with cancer fear intimacy and sex and are afraid to engage in these life-affirming activities. Rather than risking the feelings these changes arouse, some ill people, and those around them, simply withdraw. They need reassurance and help. Contact with others is a human need that never stops. Giving and receiving love can help allay fears, provide encouragement to endure treatments, and erase some of the dehumanizing effects of illness.

What can I do to help the cancer patient and myself to live with the disabilities and discouragements that go with illness?

Even when someone is extremely ill, it is important to allow them the dignity of functioning as a full participant in family life and decisions. Here are a few guidelines that may be helpful:

- Permit the person to be a decision maker. Small and large decisions and choices are made every day. Allowing the person to be part of the decision making is a good way to keep self-respect.

- Remember that the person closest to the patient may be the one who is most resented by that patient. Don't be alarmed if sometimes the ill person lashes out at you. Recognize the anger for what it is and try not to be hurt by it.
- Take especially good care of yourself. You will be of no help to anyone in this crisis if you allow yourself to bend under the strain. Plan some time each day when you can do something special for yourself.

Why, as the husband of a mastectomy patient, do I feel angrier now than when it first happened?

Your feelings are probably more commonplace than you might suspect. A Buffalo, New York, study found that many husbands whose wives had mastectomies had gone through the illness without discussing their feelings with anyone. Their initial emotional reactions were intense. They were afraid that their wives might die or that they might not be able to offer enough emotional support to them through the crisis. All the men said they had talked with their wives about her concerns over breast loss and dying, but none had talked through their own fears and worries. This behavior, it was found, led to several problems. Trying to be calm and unruffled when with their wives made the men more stressed and moody. They reported loss of energy and growing fears about their own health and death. Their lack of communication also complicated discussions with their wives about such issues as sexual adjustment and fear of death. Moreover, the wives did not believe their husbands' facade of self-assurance and became distrustful and resentful.

It was shown that a support group for the husbands helped them to disclose their fears about the possibility of losing their wives as well as highlighting their personal strengths and weaknesses and feelings of guilt. The men reported that the support group also helped them to see how their denials were complicating their emotional and marital lives rather than aiding them.

Is it a good idea for parents of children with cancer to become involved in self-help groups?

Self-help groups are structured for many specific categories (see Chapter 3). They can provide you with medical information, contacts with other people whose problems are similar to yours, various kinds of social and emotional support, as well as practical assistance. Even though every experience is different, other people can be helpful because they understand the situation as neither your doctor nor your old friends can. The self-help group can set the focus on thinking and adapting realistically and positively, giving you an opportunity to reconsider and evaluate your feelings and attitudes.

Is it wise for us to plan a vacation trip while the patient is still under treatment?

We have known many people who have gone off on extended trips—sailing, touring, archeological digs, or just beach-sitting—and regained their sense of themselves. It's fine as long as you make preparations. The first step is to talk with the doctor. Find out whether there is one time during treatment that is better for the patient to be away. Find out how long the person can be away from treatment or whether treatment can be given at another location. You will need to know:

- How to get in touch with the doctor if there is a problem.
- The name, address, and phone numbers of doctors who are experienced in the treatment in the areas where you will be traveling.
- How to register in advance at an out-of-town hospital or office, what their routine is, how the treatment will be done. It is unwise just to show up and expect to be cared for. Be aware that routines at different hospitals and offices may vary slightly.

- What arrangements need to be made to pay for treatment. You also need to know whether the bookkeeping office will accept your insurance or whether you will have to pay for the treatment in advance.
- If it might be possible for the patient to administer the treatment for himself. Discuss with the doctor the kinds of medications you should bring with you and possible problems and side effects. Be certain to bring your medical records and treatment protocols.

What extra plans need to be made for trips overseas?

There will be a few extra precautions to take to ensure that you are prepared for all eventualities:

- Go armed with names of doctors in the countries where you will be traveling. Your own doctor is the best source for names. If your doctor cannot help, call the Cancer Information Service.
- See if the doctor is willing to teach someone in the family to give drugs if needed. Perhaps he can recommend an oral form of the medication that can be taken while on the trip.
- Check insurance coverage for overseas. Most overseas doctors will require payment even when insurance covers medical treatment.
- Check with the doctor to be certain that any required immunization shots will not interfere with other medications.
- Carry medical histories, current prognosis, and treatment regimen information with you, as well as information as to where and when your doctor can be reached if needed.

What can a family do when they've been told and are trying to prepare themselves for the death of the cancer patient and the patient recovers?

This happens more frequently than one would dare to imagine with so many new and effective treatments available, particularly in families where the diagnosis of cancer still means death. When a family member has cancer, some people begin to prepare themselves for what they consider is the inevitable. In so doing, they may unconsciously begin excluding the patient from family life and decisions, in a way "practicing" what it will be like when the person dies. When the patient recovers, there can be unexpected resentment leading to feelings of guilt and remorse on the part of both the patient and other family members. It's important not to allow yourself to get into this double bind. Being aware that this can happen, you should discuss it with family members, help each other to be realistic about the patient's outlook, and guard against making assumptions about the future.

Some Suggestions on What to Say

Try saying:
- I love you because you're you.
- I'm here for you.
- I'll always be here for you.
- I'll help in any way I can, any time, at your convenience.
- I'll be thinking of you (and praying for you).
- It's hard, I know.
- I see you as a TRIUMPHER.

Don't say:
- I know *exactly* how you feel. (Unless you've been there, you don't.)
- I have a friend who's going through the same thing, only worse.
- I saw in the paper that they're curing cancer in Mexico (or Germany, etc.).
- I feel as bad about this as you do.
- I don't want to hear about cancer anymore. I've had too many friends die.
- It's just God's will and you can't do anything about it.

Avoid these platitudes:
- After all, we're all terminal.
- I could be run over by a car tomorrow.
- Do what your doctors say, they know best.
- We don't understand it, but we have to accept it.
- It could happen to any of us.
- My friend who's younger than you had an even worse case.
- Be glad you're alive.
- You're going to be just fine.

chapter 9

Where to Get Help

Although the information given in this chapter is as up-to-date as possible, the field of cancer is dynamic and constantly changing. You should expect to find that some of your inquiries will be routed to different organizations or individuals and that you should not limit your investigations to the organizations listed here.

Where is the best place to start to get help?

There are two major sources of information: The Cancer Information Service, which is supported by the National Cancer Institute, and the American Cancer Society.

What is the Cancer Information Service?

The Cancer Information Service (CIS) is a nationwide toll-free telephone service (1-800-4-CANCER), funded in many areas by the National Cancer Institute. A trained staff answers (or will find answers to) questions for the general public, in layman's language, and for health professionals. The staff can give you information on causes of cancer, how to help prevent it, methods of detection, how cancer is diagnosed, ways of treatment, rehabilitation assistance, medical facilities, home-care assistance programs, financial aids, emotional counseling services, and patient referrals. It can provide support, understanding, and rapid access to the latest information on cancer and local resources. It can tell you where in the country investigational treatment is being conducted, using PDQ, a computerized database of the National Cancer Institute. CIS can tell you what hospitals and doctors in your area are involved in what kinds of investigational treatment. If, for instance, a relative lives in a different part of the country, the staff can get information on treatment in that area. In many places, the Cancer Information Service offices are affiliated with Comprehensive Cancer Centers (specialized research and treatment centers designated by the National Cancer Institute) and with the American Cancer Society.

What kind of questions should I ask when I call the Cancer Information Service?

The more specific you can be with your questions, especially the type and stage of cancer (ask your doctor for this information), the better the information you will receive. It is wise to think through what you want to know and to write down the questions you want to have answered before you call. You can call as many times as you wish. You do not have to give your name if you do not want to. All calls are kept confidential.

Can the Cancer Information Service send me written information about cancer?

The Cancer Information Service offices are supplied with a wealth of printed information about cancer. All of them have brochures supplied by the National Cancer Institute. Some also have available brochures from the American Cancer Society. The material will be sent to you free of charge.

How can I call the Cancer Information Service?

By dialing the easy-to-remember number: 1-800-4-CANCER (1-800-422-6237). The Cancer Information Service covers the entire United States. You will be connected to the regional center that covers your area, based on the area code from which you are dialing. On Oahu, call 524-1234; neighboring islands can call collect.

Can I call the Cancer Information Service at any time?

In the majority of offices, service is on a 9:00 A.M.-to-4:30 P.M. basis. After regular hours (until 9:00 P.M. Eastern time) and on Saturdays until 6:00 P.M., callers are routed to the central office at the National Cancer Institute.

What is PDQ?

PDQ, which stands for Physician Data Query, is a computer system that gives up-to-date information on treatment for over 80 types of cancer. It is a service of the National Cancer Institute for doctors and for people with cancer and their families. PDQ tells about the current treatments for most cancers. The information in PDQ is reviewed each month by cancer experts and is updated when there is new information. PDQ also tells about clinical trials (research on treatments) and lists doctors who treat cancer and hospitals with cancer programs.

How can I get information from PDQ?

You can call the Cancer Information Service (1-800-4-CANCER) to get the latest information. Ask the staff member to do a PDQ search for you. Their trained counselors use many information resources, including PDQ, to help patients. In order to get a PDQ search, you will need to know the stage of disease, the type of cancer, and the area of the country where you are willing to go for treatment. When you get the PDQ information, you will need to bring it to your doctor, who knows you and has the facts about your disease and can help advise which treatment would be best for you.

What is the National Cancer Institute?

The National Cancer Institute (NCI) is the federal government's principal agency for research on cancer prevention, diagnosis, treatment, and rehabilitation, and for dissemination of information for the control of cancer. The Institute is one of 11 research institutes and 4 divisions that form the National Institutes of Health, located in Bethesda, Maryland. As an agency of the Department of Health and Human Services, the NCI receives annual appropriations from Congress. These funds support cancer research in the Institute's Bethesda headquarters and in about 1,000 laboratories and medical centers throughout the United States. The director of the NCI is Samuel Broder, M.D. The address is National Cancer Institute, National Institutes of Health, Bethesda, MD 20892.

Where are the Comprehensive Cancer Centers located?

There are 20 Comprehensive Cancer Centers designated by the National Cancer Institute. These medical research centers investigate new methods of diagnosis and treatment of cancer patients and provide new scientific knowledge to doctors who are treating cancer patients. They must meet 10 specific criteria, which include basic and clinical research and patient care. Comprehensive Cancer Centers have teams of experts working together on problems of research, teaching, and patient care. They treat cancer patients, will give second opinions on treatments, and try new treatments to see if they are more effective than the standard ones. They are knowledgeable about the latest developments in cancer treatment.

ALABAMA
University of Alabama
  Comprehensive Cancer
  Center
1918 University Boulevard,
Room 108
Birmingham, AL 35294
205-934-6612

CALIFORNIA
Kenneth Norris, Jr.,
  Comprehensive Cancer
  Center
Kenneth Norris, Jr., Cancer
  Hospital and Research
  Institute
University of Southern
  California
1441 Eastlake Avenue
Los Angeles, CA 90033-0804
213-226-2370

Jonsson Comprehensive
  Cancer Center
UCLA Medical Center
10-247 Factor Building
10833 Le Conte Avenue
Los Angeles, CA 90024-1781
213-825-8727

CONNECTICUT
Yale University
  Comprehensive Cancer
  Center
333 Cedar Street
New Haven, CT 06510
203-785-6338

DISTRICT OF COLUMBIA
Howard University Cancer
  Research Center
2041 Georgia Avenue, NW
Washington, DC 20060
202-636-7610 or 636-5665

Vincent T. Lombardi Cancer
  Research Center
Georgetown University
  Medical Center
3800 Reservoir Road, NW
Washington, DC 20007
202-687-2110

FLORIDA
Sylvester Comprehensive
  Cancer Center
University of Miami Medical
  School
1475 Northwest 12th Avenue
Miami, FL 33136
305-548-4850

ILLINOIS
Illinois Cancer Council
(Includes institutions listed
and several other
organizations)

Illinois Cancer Council
36 South Wabash Avenue
Chicago, IL 60603
312-226-2371

University of Chicago Cancer
  Research Center
5841 South Maryland
  Avenue
Chicago, IL 60637
312-702-9200

MARYLAND
The Johns Hopkins Oncology
  Center
600 North Wolfe Street
Baltimore, MD 21205
301-955-8638

MASSACHUSETTS
Dana-Farber Cancer
  Institute
44 Binney Street
Boston, MA 02115
617-732-3214

MICHIGAN
Meyer L. Prentis
  Comprehensive Cancer
  Center of Metropolitan
  Detroit
110 East Warren Street
Detroit, MI 48201
313-745-4329

MINNESOTA
Mayo Comprehensive
  Cancer Center
Mayo Clinic
200 First Street, SW
Rochester, MN 55905
507-284-3413

NEW YORK
Memorial Sloan-Kettering
  Cancer Center
1275 York Avenue
New York, NY 10021
1-800-525-2225

Columbia University Cancer
  Center
College of Physicians and
  Surgeons
630 West 168th Street
New York, NY 10032
212-305-6730

Roswell Park Memorial
  Institute
666 Elm Street
Buffalo, NY 14263
716-845-4400

NORTH CAROLINA
Duke University
  Comprehensive Cancer
  Center
P.O. Box 3843
Durham, NC 27710
919-286-5515

OHIO
Ohio State University
    Comprehensive Cancer
    Center
410 West 12th Avenue
Columbus, OH 43210
614-293-8619

PENNSYLVANIA
Fox Chase Cancer Center
7701 Burholme Avenue
Philadelphia, PA 19111
215-728-2570

University of Pennsylvania
    Cancer Center
3400 Spruce Street
Philadelphia, PA 19104
215-662-6364

TEXAS
The University of Texas
    M.D. Anderson Cancer
    Center
1515 Holcombe Boulevard
Houston, TX 77030
713-792-3245

WASHINGTON
Fred Hutchinson Cancer
    Research Center
1124 Columbia Street
Seattle, WA 98104
206-467-4675

WISCONSIN
Wisconsin Clinical Cancer
    Center
University of Wisconsin
600 Highland Avenue
Madison, WI 53792
608-263-6872

What are Clinical Cancer Centers?

Clinical Cancer Centers are medical centers which have support from the National Cancer Institute for programs to investigate promising new methods of cancer diagnosis and treatment.

ARIZONA
University of Arizona Cancer
    Center
1501 North Campbell
    Avenue
Tucson, AZ 85724
602-626-6372

CALIFORNIA
City of Hope National
    Medical Center
Beckman Research Institute
1500 East Duarte Road
Duarte, CA 91010
818-359-8111, ext. 2292

University of California at
San Diego Cancer Center
225 Dickinson Street
San Diego, CA 92103
619-543-6178

Charles R. Drew University
of Medicine and Science
(consortium)
12714 South Avalon
Boulevard, Suite 301
Los Angeles, CA 90061
213-603-3120

Northern California Cancer
Center (consortium)
1301 Shoreway Road
Belmont, CA 94002
415-591-4484

COLORADO
University of Colorado
Cancer Center
4200 East 9th Avenue, Box
B190
Denver, CO 80262
303-270-3019

KENTUCKY
Lucille Parker Markey
Cancer Center
University of Kentucky
Medical Center
800 Rose Street
Lexington, KY 40536
606-257-4447

MICHIGAN
University of Michigan
Cancer Center
101 Simpson Drive
Ann Arbor, MI 48109-0752
313-936-2516

NEW HAMPSHIRE
Norris Cotton Cancer Center
Dartmouth-Hitchcock
Medical Center
2 Maynard Street
Hanover, NH 03756
603-646-5505

NEW YORK
Mt. Sinai School of Medicine
1 Gustave L. Levy Place
New York, NY 10029
212-241-8617

Albert Einstein College of
Medicine
1300 Morris Park Avenue
Bronx, NY 10461
212-920-4826

New York University Cancer
Center
462 First Avenue
New York, NY 10016
212-340-6485

University of Rochester
Cancer Center
601 Elmwood Avenue, Box
704
Rochester, NY 14642
716-275-4911

NORTH CAROLINA
Lineberger Cancer Research
  Center
University of North Carolina
  School of Medicine
Chapel Hill, NC 27599
919-966-4431

Bowman Gray School of
  Medicine
Wake Forest University
300 South Hawthorne Road
Winston-Salem, NC 27103
919-748-4354

OHIO
Case Western Reserve
  University
University Hospitals of
  Cleveland
Ireland Cancer Center
2074 Abington Road
Cleveland, OH 44106
216-844-8453

PENNSYLVANIA
Pittsburgh Cancer Institute
230 Lothrop Street
Pittsburgh, PA 15213-2592
1-800-537-4063

RHODE ISLAND
Roger Williams General
  Hospital
825 Chalkstone Avenue
Providence, RI 02908
401-456-2070

TENNESSEE
St. Jude Children's Research
  Hospital
332 North Lauderdale Street
Memphis, TN 38101
901-522-0694

UTAH
Utah Regional Cancer Center
University of Utah Medical
  Center
50 North Medical Drive,
  Room 2C10
Salt Lake City, UT 84132
801-581-4048

VERMONT
Vermont Regional Cancer
  Center
University of Vermont
1 South Prospect Street
Burlington, VT 05401
802-656-4580

VIRGINIA
Massey Cancer Center
Medical College of Virginia
Virginia Commonwealth
  University
1200 East Broad Street
Richmond, VA 23298
804-786-9641

University of Virginia
  Medical Center
Box 334
Primary Care Center, Rm 4520
Lee Street
Charlottesville, VA 22908
804-924-2562

Where are clinical cooperative groups located?

Clinical cooperative groups, funded by the National Cancer
Institute to investigate promising new methods of cancer
treatment, are located in many of the medical institutions in
the United States and abroad. Some 4,000 cancer-research
physicians in the United States and overseas are involved.
Following laboratory research, the treatment under study is
evaluated in cancer patients. Information on the clinical cooperative groups, the kinds of cancer being studied, and
physicians who are located near your home can be obtained
by calling the Cancer Information Service.

What are community clinical oncology programs?

The National Cancer Institute has funded over 50 community clinical oncology programs (CCOPs) in states around the
country, at community hospitals, or groups of community
cancer specialists. The program is designed to combine the
expertise of community doctors with ongoing research
projects and to introduce the newest clinical research findings into community settings. Qualified community physicians participate in clinical trials by affiliating with treatment
study programs at major medical centers and national and
regional clinical cooperative groups that conduct large treatment studies. You can get information on what doctors in
your area are involved in clinical trials by calling the Cancer
Information Service at 1-800-4-CANCER.

**What is the National Cancer Institute's clinical treatment
program?**

The National Cancer Institute is studying new treatments at
the National Institutes of Health's Clinical Center in Bethesda, Maryland. To learn whether a cancer patient is eligible to

participate in a research study at the Clinical Center, the patient's doctor may send a complete medical report to the Deputy Clinical Director, National Cancer Institute, Building 10, Room 6B15, Bethesda, MD 20892. The telephone number for physician referrals is 301-496-4251.

What is the American Cancer Society?

The American Cancer Society (ACS), a voluntary organization of some 2.5 million Americans, is a national organization fighting cancer through research, education, and patient service and rehabilitation programs. It is composed of a national society with 57 chartered divisions and nearly 3,000 local units. The national society administers programs of research, medical grants, and clinical fellowships and is charged with carrying out public and professional education at the national level. The divisions are in all states, in addition to six metropolitan areas, the District of Columbia, and Puerto Rico. The units are organized to cover the counties in the United States. Some units have branches which cover smaller geographic areas.

What kind of help can I get through the American Cancer Society?

The units of the American Cancer Society conduct basic service programs, including information and counseling services for the cancer patient and the patient's family (information and guidance concerning ACS services, community health services, and other resources), equipment loans (sickroom supplies and special comfort items to assist in caring for the homebound patient, such as hospital beds, walkers, aspirators, blenders, bedpans, urinals, pressure pillows, incontinence pads, and wheelchairs, etc.), surgical dressings prepared by volunteers, and transportation to and from a doctor's office, clinic, or hospital for treatment. Some also provide home health care, blood programs, assistance with employment problems, social-work assistance, limited financial assistance, and medications. Rehabilitation programs, primarily directed toward laryngectomy, mastectomy, and ostomy patients, are an important part of the service offered.

What are some of the support groups the Cancer Society runs?

There are several programs. Those which involve a volunteer visitor include Reach to Recovery (for women who have or had breast cancer), ostomy (for people who have a stoma as a result of colon or rectal survey), and laryngectomy (for people who have lost their voices). They also help support the Candlelighters Childhood Cancer Foundation (for parents of children with cancer), CanSurmount (which matches a volunteer who has had cancer with a patient for hospital visits), I Can Cope (a course designed to address educational and psychological needs), and summer camps for children.

How can I reach the American Cancer Society?

You can reach local units in most areas of the country by telephone. Look in the White Pages under American Cancer Society. Ask for the person in charge of patient services. The American Cancer Society can also answer many questions by telephone and offers printed material on cancer free of charge. You can also reach the Cancer Society through a toll-free number, 1-800-ACS-2345.

Will I have to visit the offices of the American Cancer Society in order to get help?

It depends upon what you are looking for. If you want counseling help or are looking for guidance in finding resources for financial aid, you will probably need to visit the office to discuss your problems. If you are looking for loan equipment, you will have to make arrangements to pick it up. If you have a simple question, it will probably be answered immediately on the phone. Your first step in all cases, however, is to make a telephone call.

What is the mailing address for the American Cancer Society?

The address for the national office is American Cancer Society, 1599 Clifton Road, NE, Atlanta, GA 30329; telephone: 404-320-3333. The addresses for the divisions are as follows:

Alabama Division, Inc.
402 Office Park Drive
Suite 300
Birmingham, AL 35223
205-879-2242

Alaska Division, Inc.
406 West Fireweed Lane
Suite 101
Anchorage, AK 99503
907-277-8696

Arizona Division, Inc.
2929 East Thomas Road
Phoenix, AZ 85016
602-224-0524

Arkansas Division, Inc.
P.O. Box 3822
Little Rock, AR 72203
501-664-3480-1-2

California Division, Inc.
1710 Webster Street
P.O. Box 2061
Oakland, CA 94612
415-893-7900

Colorado Division, Inc.
2255 South Oneida
P.O. Box 24669
Denver, CO 80224
303-758-2030

Connecticut Division, Inc.
Barnes Park South
14 Village Lane
P.O. Box 410
Wallingford, CT 06492
203-265-7161

Delaware Division, Inc.
1708 Lovering Avenue
Suite 202
Wilmington, DE 19806
302-654-6267

District of Columbia
    Division, Inc.
Universal Building, South
1825 Connecticut Avenue,
    NW
Washington, DC 20009
202-483-2600

Florida Division, Inc.
1001 South MacDill Avenue
Tampa, FL 33629
813-253-0541

Georgia Division, Inc.
46 Fifth Street, NE
Atlanta, GA 30308
404-892-0026

Hawaii Pacific Division, Inc.
Community Services Center
  Building
200 North Vineyard
  Boulevard
Honolulu, HI 96817
808-531-1662-3-4-5

Idaho Division, Inc.
1609 Abbs Street
P.O. Box 5386
Boise, ID 83705
208-343-4609

Illinois Division, Inc.
37 South Wabash Avenue
Chicago, IL 60603
312-372-0472

Indiana Division, Inc.
9575 North Valparaiso Court
Indianapolis, IN 46268
317-872-4432

Iowa Division, Inc.
8364 Hickman Road
Suite D
Des Moines, IA 50322
515-253-0147

Kansas Division, Inc.
3003 Van Buren Street
Topeka, KS 66611
913-267-0131

Kentucky Division, Inc.
Medical Arts Building
1169 Eastern Parkway
Louisville, KY 40217
502-459-1867

Louisiana Division, Inc.
Fidelity Homestead Building
837 Gravier Street
Suite 700
New Orleans, LA
  70112-1509
504-523-2029

Maine Division, Inc.
52 Federal Street
Brunswick, ME 04011
207-729-3339

Maryland Division, Inc.
8219 Town Center Drive
P.O. Box 82
White Marsh, MD
  21162-0082
301-529-7272

Massachusetts Division, Inc.
247 Commonwealth Avenue
Boston, MA 02116
617-267-2650

Michigan Division, Inc.
1205 East Saginaw Street
Lansing, MI 48906
517-371-2920

Minnesota Division, Inc.
3316 West 66th Street
Minneapolis, MN 55435
612-925-2772

Mississippi Division, Inc.
1380 Livingston Lane
Lakeover Office Park
Jackson, MS 39213
601-362-8874

Missouri Division, Inc.
3322 American Avenue
P.O. Box 1066
Jefferson City, MO 65102
314-893-4800

Montana Division, Inc.
313 North 32nd Street
Suite 1
Billings, MT 59101
406-252-7111

Nebraska Division, Inc.
8502 West Center Road
Omaha, NE 68124-5255
402-393-5800

Nevada Division, Inc.
1325 East Harmon
Las Vegas, NV 89119
702-798-6877

New Hampshire Division,
   Inc.
360 Route 101
Unit 501
Bedford, NH 03102
603-669-3270

New Jersey Division, Inc.
2600 Route 1, CNN 2201
North Brunswick, NJ 08902
201-297-8000

New Mexico Division, Inc.
5800 Lomas Boulevard, NE
Albuquerque, NM 87110
505-262-2336

New York State Division,
   Inc.
6725 Lyons Street
P.O. Box 7
East Syracuse, NY 13057
315-437-7025

   Long Island Division, Inc.
   145 Pidgeon Hill Road
   Huntington Station, NY
      11746
   516-385-9100

   New York City Division,
      Inc.
   19 West 56th Street
   New York, NY 10019
   212-586-8700

   Queens Division, Inc.
   112-25 Queens Boulevard
   Forest Hills, NY 11375
   718-263-2224

   Westchester Division, Inc.
   30 Glenn Street
   White Plains, NY 10603
   914-949-4800

North Carolina Division,
Inc.
11 South Boylan Avenue
Suite 221
Raleigh, NC 27603
919-834-8463

North Dakota Division, Inc.
Hotel Graver Annex
Building
115 Roberts Street
P.O. Box 426
Fargo, ND 58107
701-232-1385

Ohio Division, Inc.
5555 Frantz Road
Dublin, OH 43017
614-889-9565

Oklahoma Division, Inc.
300 United Founders
Boulevard
Suite 136
Oklahoma City, OK 73112
405-946-5000

Oregon Division, Inc.
0330 Southwest Curry
Portland, OR 97201
503-295-6422

Pennsylvania Division, Inc.
Route 422 & Sipe Avenue
P.O. Box 897
Hershey, PA 17033-0897
717-533-6144

Philadelphia Division, Inc.
1422 Chestnut Street
Philadelphia, PA 19102
215-665-2900

Puerto Rico Division, Inc.
Calle Alverío #577
Esquina Sargento Medina
Hato Rey, PR 00936
809-764-2295

Rhode Island Division, Inc.
400 Main Street
Pawtucket, RI 02860
401-722-8480

South Carolina Division,
Inc.
2214 Devine Street
Columbia, SC 29205
803-256-0245

South Dakota Division, Inc.
4101 Carnegie Circle
Sioux Falls, SD 57106-2322
605-336-0897

Tennessee Division, Inc.
1315 Eighth Avenue South
Nashville, TN 37203
615-255-1ACS

Texas Division, Inc.
P.O. Box 140435
Austin, TX 78714-0435
512-928-2262

Utah Division, Inc.
610 East South Temple
Salt Lake City, UT 84102
801-322-0431

Vermont Division, Inc.
13 Loomis Street, Drawer C
Montpelier, VT 05602
802-223-2348

Virginia Division, Inc.
4240 Park Place Court
P.O. Box 1547
Glen Allen, VA 23060
804-270-0142

Washington Division, Inc.
2120 First Avenue North
Seattle, WA 98109-1140
206-283-1152

West Virginia Division, Inc.
2428 Kanawha Boulevard
East Charleston, WV 25311
304-344-3611

Wisconsin Division, Inc.
615 North Sherman Avenue
Madison, WI 53704
608-249-0487

Wyoming Division, Inc.
3109 Boxelder Drive
Cheyenne, WY 82001
307-638-3331

What is the National Coalition for Cancer Survivorship?

The National Coalition for Cancer Survivorship, founded in 1986, is a network of independent groups and individuals concerned with survivorship and support of those with cancer and their loved ones. Its programs provide a national communication network, a forum for discussion of survivorship issues, advocacy to reduce cancer-based discrimination, and information and resources on life after a cancer diagnosis. The organization publishes a quarterly newsletter. You can reach the National Coalition for Cancer Survivorship at 323 Eighth Street, SW, Alburquerque, NM 87102; telephone: 505-764-9956.

Is there an organization that can help me find health information?

The National Health Information Center is a health information referral organization that puts people with health questions in touch with those organizations best able to answer them. Established in 1979 by the Office of Disease Prevention and Health Promotion of the Department of Health and Human Services, the center's main objectives are to identify health information resources, channel requests for information to these resources, and develop publications on health-related topics of interest to health professionals, the health media, and the general public. To reach the center, call toll free 1-800-336-4797; in Maryland: 301-565-4167, or write P.O. Box 1133, Washington DC 20013-1133. The center's referral specialists will search its resource files and its database to find organizations that can respond to questions and will put callers in touch with the organizations by giving toll-free numbers if available, providing callers with the organizations' full addresses and phone numbers, or referring questions to appropriate organizations so they can reply directly to requests. The center also runs the National Information Center for Orphan Drugs and Rare Diseases which responds to inquiries on rare diseases and on drugs which are not widely researched or available. The address is the same as for the National Health Center. The toll-free number is 1-800-456-3505.

What organizations are working as advocates for cancer survivors in the areas of job discrimination and similar issues?

There are several. The National Coalition on Cancer Survivorship is providing legal aid and advice on obtaining jobs.

Barbara Hoffman, a lawyer, works on advocacy issues for the coalition (609-799-9199). Grace Monaco, also a lawyer, has been a leading advocate for the rights of young cancer patients since she founded the Candlelighters Children Cancer Foundation in 1970. The American Cancer Society (Morton Bard, vice-president for services and rehabilitation at the Society's headquarters in Atlanta) has been in the forefront in the discrimination issue and has recently written the Cancer Survivors' Bill of Rights. Call 202-659-5136, or address inquiries to 1901 Pennsylvania Avenue, NW, Suite 1001, Washington DC 20006.

What is the Cancer Survivors' Bill of Rights?

The American Cancer Society has presented a Survivors' Bill of Rights to call attention to the needs of survivors and to enhance cancer care:

1. Survivors have the right to assurance of lifelong medical care, as needed. The physicians and other professionals involved in their care should continue their constant efforts to be:
   - sensitive to the cancer survivors' lifestyle choices and their need for self-esteem and dignity;
   - careful, no matter how long they have survived, to have symptoms taken seriously, and not have aches and pains dismissed, for fear of recurrence is a normal part of survivorship;
   - informative and open, providing survivors with as much or as little candid medical information as they wish, and encouraging their informed participation in their own care;
   - knowledgeable about counseling resources, and willing to refer survivors and their families as appropriate for emotional support and therapy which will improve the quality of individual lives.

2. In their personal lives, survivors, like other Americans, have the right to the pursuit of happiness. This means they have the right:

- to talk with their families and friends about their cancer experience if they wish, but to refuse to discuss it if that is their choice and not to be expected to be more upbeat or less blue than anyone else;
- to be free of the stigma of cancer as a "dread disease" in all social relations;
- to be free of blame for having gotten the disease and of guilt for having survived it.

3. In the workplace, survivors have the right to equal job opportunities. This means they have the right:

- to aspire to jobs worthy of their skills, and for which they are trained and experienced, and thus not to have to accept jobs they would not have considered before the cancer experience;
- to be hired, promoted and accepted on return to work, according to their individual abilities and qualifications, and not according to "cancer" or "disability" stereotypes;
- to privacy about their medical histories.

4. Since health insurance coverage is an overriding survivorship concern, every effort should be made to assure all survivors adequate health insurance, whether public or private. This means:

- for employers, that survivors have the right to be included in group health coverage, which is usually less expensive, provides better benefits, and covers the employee regardless of health history;
- for physicians, counselors, and other professionals concerned, that they keep themselves and their survivor-clients informed and up-to-date on available group or individual health policy options, noting, for example, what major expenses like hospital costs and medical tests outside the hospital are covered and what amount must be paid before coverage (deductibles).

What is Make Today Count?

Make Today Count is an organization which gives emotional support to patients with cancer or with any other life-threatening illness. Their main aim is to help people live every day as fully and as happily as possible. They have activities such as group meetings, home visits, and educational workshops, as well as newsletters and other informational materials.

Make Today Count was founded in 1974 and has some 135 chapters throughout the United States and in several foreign countries. Look in your phone book to see if there is a local chapter or write to Make Today Count, Inc., 101½ South Union Street, Alexandria, VA 22314-3348; telephone: 703-548-9674 or 703-548-9714.

Is there a special organization for people who have lost their voices as a result of cancer?

There is such an organization: the International Association of Laryngectomees (IAL), composed of member clubs. It gives information and education both before and after the operation to people who have lost their voices. You can get a list of speech instructors and educational materials from them. In some areas, they will also send out another cancer patient who has had the same problem. The organization is sponsored by the American Cancer Society. For more information, contact the local office of the Cancer Society or the Office of the Program Associate Director of IAL at 1599 Clifton Road, NE, Atlanta, GA 30392; telephone: 404-320-3333.

What is Reach to Recovery?

Reach to Recovery helps breast cancer patients with their physical, emotional, and cosmetic needs. Trained volunteer visitors provide support and information before and after the operation. Hospital visits are made at the request of your doctor. (If your doctor does not mention it, ask him or the nurse to make arrangements for a visit. Or you can call the American Cancer Society directly when you get home from the hospital.) Reach to Recovery also can give information and literature on post-operation exercises, and on where to find a certain prosthesis or different kinds of prostheses. It is a program of the American Cancer Society.

What is Encore?

Encore is a discussion and exercise program for women who have had breast cancer surgery. It is run by the YWCA and includes exercising to music, water exercises, and discussion. A woman may join the group the third week after surgery, with written permission from her doctor. Call your local YWCA for additional information or write to Encore, National Board, YWCA, 726 Broadway, New York, NY 10003; telephone: 212-614-2827.

What is CanSurmount?

CanSurmount is a patient visitor program which matches medically stabilized and successfully adjusted cancer patients with other cancer patients for a one-to-one limited-term visitation program. The volunteer visitors provide emotional support and an outlet for patients to voice fears and anxieties. The program was begun over a decade ago in Denver, Colorado, by a medical oncologist, Paul Hamilton, M.D., and his patient, Lynne Ringer, who recognized that those who have had cancer may be uniquely qualified to understand the concerns, fears, and frustrations of other cancer patients. The program is specifically tailored to the needs of the individuals. CanSurmount is a program of the American Cancer Society and can be reached by calling your local American Cancer Society office.

Is there some help for people who have a stoma as a result of an operation for colon or rectal cancer?

Yes, there is. The United Ostomy Association is organized and administered by people with ostomies. It helps people return to a normal life after an ostomy operation through mutual aid and emotional support. There are some 700 local chapters throughout the country. The organization supports the improvement of ostomy equipment and supplies and publishes the *Ostomy Quarterly* and other educational materials. In addition, your doctor can ask for a volunteer from the association who will visit with new ostomy patients. For additional information, look in your phone book or write to 36 Executive Park, Suite 120, Irvine, CA 92714; telephone: 714-660-8624.

The American Cancer Society also has an ostomy rehabilitation program. In many areas it is affiliated with the United Ostomy Association. Check your phone book and call the local American Cancer Society unit for further information. Or contact the American Cancer Society national headquarters, 1599 Clifton Road, NE, Atlanta, GA 30329; telephone: 404-320-3333.

What is the Candelighters Childhood Cancer Foundation?

This is an organization formed by parents of young cancer patients. It helps families cope with the emotional stresses of their experience. Candelighters holds regular meetings to discuss problems and to exchange information, distributes free newsletters for young people and adults, stimulates local interest in the special concerns of young people with cancer, and works to gain support for programs of cancer research in this area.

Candelighters was started in 1970 and has some 225 parent groups throughout the world. Since 1977, it has been supported in part by the American Cancer Society. For further information, check your local phone book or write to Candlelighters Foundation, 1901 Pennsylvania Avenue, NW, Suite 1001, Washington, DC 20006; telephone: 202-659-5136.

What is the Association for the Care of Children's Health?

Founded in 1965, the Association for the Care of Children's Health is a non-profit, international organization of over 4,000 members representing parents and health professionals. It carries out a variety of programs to promote the health and well-being of children and their families in all health-care settings. The association works to meet the emotional and developmental needs of children and families through education and research, in addition to helping develop federal guidelines about child patient care. It also publishes educational materials. The association is located at 3615 Wisconsin Avenue, NW, Washington, DC 20016; telephone: 202-244-1801.

What is Hospice?

Hospice is a program that offers care for terminally ill patients and provides supportive services for family members. It recognizes that dying people and their families have needs that are different from those of people with curable diseases and has programs designed for these special needs. In a hospice, controlling pain and symptoms are main concerns, so patients can be as alert and as comfortable as possible.

There are many different kinds of hospice programs. Some offer home care, some offer care in a hospice center, some are in a hospital or in a skilled nursing facility. Many offer a combination of services within a single program.

For many people, part of hospice expenses may be paid by health insurance plans, either group policies offered by employers or individual policies. Ask a hospital social worker, your company's personnel office, or your insurance company to give you information about your own situation. Your Medicare or Medicaid insurance may also provide payment.

To find out information about hospices in your area, you may call the Cancer Information Service at 1-800-4-CANCER. Or contact Hospicelink at 1-800-331-1620 (5 Essex Square, P.O. Box 713, Essex, CT 06426) or the National Hospice Organization, 1901 North Fort Myer Drive, Suite 901, Arlington, VA 22209; telephone: 703-243-5900. This organization can provide information about services in different areas. There is also an agency which encourages use of hospices and home-care programs for children called Children's Hospice International, 1101 King Street, Suite 131, Alexandria, VA 22314; telephone: 703-684-0330.

Is there a special organization for people with brain tumors?

The Association for Brain Tumor Research is a voluntary organization which supports research, promotes the understanding of brain tumors, and offers printed materials that deal with research and treatment of brain tumors. You can reach it at 3725 North Talman Avenue, Chicago, IL 60618; telephone: 312-286-5571.

Is there special help for people with leukemia or lymphoma?

There is a special organization, the Leukemia Society of America, a national voluntary health agency which provides financial assistance to patients with leukemia, the lymphomas, and Hodgkin's disease. It will also give you referrals to other sources of help in the community. The program is administered through society chapters located throughout the United States. Payment can be made for drugs used in care, treatment, and/or control of the disease, for transfusing blood, transportation to and from a doctor's office, hospital, or treatment center, and X-ray treatment.

Through its Patient Aid program, the Leukemia Society has developed local family support groups at a number of offices throughout the country. The groups are free of charge and open to patients, their families, and friends. They are intended to provide information and support, as well as to encourage greater communication among patients, their families, friends, and medical personnel. Supplementary financial assistance up to $750 a year per person is given by the society to outpatients being treated for leukemia, the lymphomas, multiple myeloma, and preleukemia. Look in your local phone book for information or call the Cancer Information Service. You can also write the Leukemia Society at 733 Third Avenue, New York, NY 10017; telephone: 212-573-8484.

What is the American Lung Association?

The American Lung Association is a voluntary organization committed to the prevention and control of lung disease. It has nearly 150 affiliates which distribute printed materials on the effects of smoking, air pollution, and occupational exposures, as well as on lung cancer. It also offers programs to encourage smokers to quit through self-help, group, and home video programs. To find the local office, look in the White Pages of your telephone directory. The national office is located at 1740 Broadway, New York, NY 10019.

What does Cancer Care do?

Cancer Care is a non-profit social service agency which helps patients and families cope with the emotional, psychological, and financial consequences of cancer. Appointments may be made for financial counseling. There is no charge for individual, family, or group counseling. Appropriate, supplementary financial assistance toward the cost of home care and transportation is available. For information, call 212-221-3300, or write Cancer Care, 1180 Avenue of the Americas, New York, NY 10036.

What is the American Kidney Fund?

The American Kidney Fund is a non-profit, national voluntary organization which provides direct financial assistance to those with kidney disease. Funds are given directly to patients. Special dietary needs, medications, home dialysis supplies, insurance, Medicare premiums, transportation costs, and other expenses related to kidney conditions may also be covered. Contact the American Kidney Fund by calling 1-800-638-8299 or 301-986-1444, or by writing 7315 Wisconsin Avenue, Bethesda, MD 20814-3266.

What is the service for men with potency problems?

There is an 800 number you can call (1-800-835-7667), a service of Grace Hospital in Detroit, Michigan, and affiliated with 23 hospitals nationwide, which provides referrals to self-help support groups and other agencies. You can also get written materials from this office.

How can I get help in transporting a patient to a major cancer center?

The Corporate Angel Network is a service that offers available space on corporate airplanes to cancer patients in need of transportation to treatment centers. It is located at the Westchester County Airport, Building 1, White Plains, NY 10604; telephone: 914-328-1313.

Are there special Outward Bound programs for cancer patients?

Yes there are. The North Carolina Outward Bound School (121 North Sterling Street, Morganton, NC 28655-3443; telephone: 704-437-6112), an internationally recognized wilderness program, offers five-day courses especially designed for cancer patients. The Colorado Outward Bound program in Denver (303-837-0880) offers weekend courses for cancer patients, friends, and relatives with cancer and health professionals. They are co-sponsored by the CanSurmount program at two Denver hospitals. The Outward Bound School in Rockland Maine (207-594-5548) offers courses for cancer patients directly as well as working with private groups to offer programs for group members.

The courses are built on the belief that individuals, through challenge and shared adventure, develop self-reliance, respect for others, and, most important, a sense of compassion. These courses have been developed especially for individuals with cancer. They are built on the key elements of the Outward Bound experience of allowing participants to challenge their physical and emotional limitations through simulated life-threatening experiences. The purpose is to increase self-confidence and encourage students to trust themselves and others. Costs vary, with some programs offering scholarship aid.

What kind of activities are offered in the Outward Bound cancer courses?

The activities include rock climbing, rappeling, wilderness hiking, camping and cooking, running, and negotiating military obstacle courses built from ropes and cargo nets. The activities are chosen to meet the needs, objectives, and abilities of the participants. The instructor chooses activities that are challenging, require group cooperation and support, and which can lead to well-earned success. There is time for learning, sharing of feelings, reflection, laughter, and play. Your fears are revealed and you find out how to function even when you're afraid.

What is the Cancer Self-Help Intensive?

The Cancer Self-Help Intensive is a long, arduous program to teach people to get in touch with the emotions they may have blocked within themselves. People attend either one seven-hour session a week for nine weeks or five days a week for two weeks—a commitment of over 60 hours of group work and skill learning. The sessions are emotion-packed, tackling topics such as life goals, family dynamics, using illness as a benefit and excuse, and death and dying. The afternoons are set aside for learning meditation, relaxation, goal setting, and visualization techniques. The Cancer Self-Help Intensive is part of the Cancer Support and Education Center in Menlo Park, California. Center director Maggie Creighton recommends the program as an adjunct to conventional treatment. The program costs $1,850, but there are scholarships, grants, and payment plans available.

What is the We Can Weekend program?

It is a weekend retreat, organized by the staff of the North Memorial Medical Center in Minneapolis and held twice a year. The two-day meeting is designed to help cancer patients and their families identify and cope with the impact the disease has on their lives. The We Can Weekend was developed because of the need for entire families to be involved in a disease which disrupts all aspects of a family's existence.

The lively weekend offers the adults a variety of workshops, including sessions on facts and fallacies about cancer, cancer treatment, stress management, massage, art therapy, and spiritual needs. School-age children spend time playing games and working on artwork that helps them to discuss their feelings. The teenagers talk with each other or play games, whatever they feel they need. There is a staff of volunteers—nurses, chaplains, CanSurmount support program counselors, art and music therapists—to help run the weekend.

You can get information on the weekend, including its local availability, by calling the North Cancer Center at 612-520-5155. Materials on how to organize a We Can Weekend retreat are available from the North Cancer Center, North Memorial Medical Center, 3300 Oakdale North, Robbinsdale, MN 55422.

How can I have our family history checked to see if we are susceptible to hereditary cancer?

The Hereditary Cancer Institute, a non-profit organization established in Nebraska in 1984, is devoted solely to the study of the genetics of familial cancer. Signals which might suggest that your family is unusually susceptible include:
- Cancer occurring at an early age
- Appearance of cancer in a close relative
- More than one cancer in a close relative
- More than one generation affected

The Institute attempts to assess and verify the nature of cancer patterns in such families in search of simple or complex modes of inheritance which may aid in predicting cancer risk to family members and their offspring. The group maintains a registry of all such families. They are seeking those who feel they might be in a cancer-risk family. If you send them your name and address, they will send you educational material, including a 12-page legal-sized single-spaced questionnaire to be filled out by you, possibly with help from your family physicians for the more medically oriented questions. Further follow-up is done, if your permission is given, through hospital and physician records. For information, contact Hereditary Cancer Institute, Creighton University, Omaha, NE 68178.

What is the National Coalition for Cancer Survivorship?

The National Coalition for Cancer Survivorship is a network of independent groups and individuals concerned with survivorship and support of cancer survivors and their loved ones (323 Eighth Street, SW, Alburquerque, NM 87102; telephone: 505-764-9956). According to Fitzhugh Mullan, a doctor and cancer survivor who is its president, it is a network for the nation's five million people who have had cancer and are living and surviving.

Mullan discusses what he calls the "seasons of survival." According to him there are three, beginning with "acute survival," which is the time of diagnosis and treatment. He feels people are fearful and anxious during this time. The second phase, "extended survival," is a period when people have completed their treatment or go into remission and enter a phase of "watchful waiting," in which they go back into the healthy world and are usually fearful of recurrence. The last season is "permanent survival." Mullan feels that people who have come through a cancer experience are indelibly affected by it—it is something that leaves people with an impression both physically and emotionally.

What are Ronald McDonald Houses?

Ronald McDonald Houses offer a home away from home for parents and families of children being treated for a serious illness. They can be found in over 60 cities in the United States and Canada and in some places overseas. Each Ronald McDonald House is different, created by teams of concerned local citizens to meet the needs of their own communities. Each House is owned and operated by a local not-for-profit organization comprised of volunteers and is primarily funded by local contributions. To contact the organization directly, write to Ronald McDonald Houses, National Coordinator, Golin Communications, Inc., 500 North Michigan Avenue, Chicago, IL 60611; telephone: 312-836-7100.

Where are camps located which serve children with cancer or their brothers or sisters?

There are many around the country. Check with your doctor to see if the camp is right for your child.

ALABAMA
CAMP RAP-A-HOPE
Contact: Lynn Fondren/Pam Koch, Directors, Camp Rap-A-Hope, P.O. Box 850872, Mobile, AL 36685. Sponsored by Mobile County Medical Society and Auxiliary. One week residential camp for children with cancer. Free.

CAMP SMILE-A-MILE
Contact: Vikki Grodner, Camp Director, P.O. Box 550155, Birmingham, AL 35255. 205-930-0119. Three one-week overnight sessions for children 5–18 with cancer or in remission from cancer. Free.

ARIZONA
CAMP SUNRISE
Contact: American Cancer Society, Manager of Childhood Cancer Services, 2929 East Thomas Road, Phoenix, AZ 85016. One-week program for children 7–15, day camps for 3–7-year-olds who have or have had cancer and their siblings in Tucson and Phoenix. Three-day sibling camp for children 11–15. Two teen weeks for ages 13–17. Transportation provided. Free.

CALIFORNIA
CAMP OKIZU
Contact: Coral Cotten, Executive Director, Robert J. Sturhahn Foundation, 2171 Francisco Boulevard, Suite L, San Rafael, CA 94901. 415-485-0872. Three programs: two-week oncology camp for children with leukemia, other cancers, or any life-threatening illness; two-week siblings camp; and three family camp weekends.

CAMP REACH FOR THE SKY—DAY CAMP
Contact: Deborah Hoffman, American Cancer Society, 2251 San Diego Avenue, Suite B-150, San Diego, CA 92110. 619-299-4200. Five-day day camp in San Diego for children 4–8, resident camp in Julian for children 8–18.

CAMP RONALD McDONALD FOR GOOD TIMES
Contact: Camp Ronald McDonald for Good Times, 520 South Sepulveda Boulevard, Suite 208, Los Angeles, CA 90049. 213-476-8488. Resident camping program for children with cancer.

CAMP SUNSHINE AND DREAMS
Contact: Joan Michelson, American Cancer Society, Fresno Unit, 2940 North Fresno Street, Fresno, CA 93703.

CAMP SUNBURST
Contact: Geri Brooks, PhD, Executive Camp Director, Columbia Pacific University Foundation, 148 Wilson Hill Road, Petaluma, CA 94952. 707-763-4782. Ten-day summer residential program for life-threatened children 6–19.

CAMP SUMMER SAULT, AMERICAN CANCER SOCIETY
Contact: Ellie Margolin, 936 Pine Avenue, Long Beach, CA 90801. 213-437-0791. Five-day day camp for children with cancer and their siblings 6–13. Leadership experience for teenagers 14 and over. Free.

COLORADO
CAMP SKY HIGH HOPE
Contact: Nancy King, RN, Camp Director, 2430 East Arkansas Avenue, Denver, CO 80218. 303-832-2667. One-week camp for children 8–17 who have or have had cancer.

CONNECTICUT
CAMP RISING SUN
Contact: Jane Bemis, American Cancer Society, CT Division, Inc., P.O. Box 410, Wallingford, CT 06492. 203-265-7161. One-week overnight program for young people 7–17 with cancer, on or off treatment. Counselor in training program for 16–17 year olds. Free.

THE HOLE-IN-THE-WALL GANG CAMP

Contact: Howard A. Pearson, MD, or Paul Newman, The Hole-in-the-Wall Gang Camp, 246 Post Road East, Westport, CT 06880. 203-222-0136. For children 7–17 under treatment for or cured of cancer, leukemia, and other major blood diseases. Four resident one-week sessions. Free.

FLORIDA
CAMP R.O.C.K.
(REACHING OUT TO CANCER KIDS)

Contact: Beverly Deason, Director of Service & Rehabilitation, American Cancer Society, FL Division, Inc., 1001 South MacDill Avenue, Tampa, FL 33629. 813-253-0541. Two one-week overnight camps for children 6–18.

GEORGIA
CAMP RAINBOW

Contact: Frances Friedman, Play Therapy, Children's Clinic for Cancer and Blood Diseases. (CK-146), MCG Hospital & Clinics, Augusta, GA 30912-3730.

CAMP SUNSHINE

Contact: Camp Sunshine, P.O. Box 77236, Atlanta, GA 30309. 404-872-6977. One-week camp for Georgian children and adolescents who have or have had leukemia or other cancers. Year-round activities, April family weekend. $50.00 donation requested but not required.

HAWAII
CAMP ANUENUE

(Hawaiian for rainbow)
Contact: Grace Y. Iwahashi, Director of Medical Affairs, American Cancer Society, HI Pacific Division, Inc., 200 North Vineyard Boulevard, Honolulu, HI 96817. For cancer patients and the physically disabled 7–14 on or off therapy and cured. Free.

IDAHO
CAMP RAINBOW GOLD

Contact: American Cancer Society, ID Division, Inc. P.O. Box 5386, Boise, ID 83705. 208-343-4609. For children 6–18 with cancer. Free.

ILLINOIS
CAMP ONE STEP AT A TIME

Contact: Edward S. Baum,

MD, or Annjeanette Laster, Division of Hematology/Oncology, Children's Memorial Hospital, 2300 Children's Plaza, Chicago, IL 60614. Two one-week overnight sessions for children with cancer from Illinois or Wisconsin.

CAMP RAINBOWS & UNICORNS

Contact: Colleen Fitzgerald, Maine-Niles Association of Special Recreation, 7640 Main Street, Niles, IL 60648. 312-966-5522. Day camp for children with cancer and their siblings 4–11. Financial aid.

INDIANA
CAMP LITTLE RED DOOR

Contact: Marion County Cancer Society, Inc., 1801 North Meridian Street, Indianapolis, IN 46202. 317-925-5595. One-week camp for children 8–18 with cancer. $75.00; financial assistance; wheelchair accessible.

IOWA
CAMP-A-PANDA

Contact: JoAnn Zimmerman, Camp Director, Camp-A-Panda, 4116 65th Street, Des Moines, IA 50322. 515-279-5444. One-week residential camp for children with cancer 5–17. Free.

KANSAS
CAMP HOPE

Contact: Jeri Heycock, Vice President of Medical Affairs, American Cancer Society, KS Division, Inc., 3003 Van Buren, Topeka, KS 66611. One-week camp for 75 children 8–18 who have or have had cancer. Free.

KENTUCKY
INDIAN SUMMER CAMP

Contact: Gloria Sams, Regional Coordinator, McDowell Cancer Network, First Federal Building, Rm. 213, 107 South Main Street, Somerset, KY 42501. 606-679-7204. One-week summer program for children 7–17 with cancer.

MAINE
CAMP RAINBOW

Contact: Camp Rainbow, American Cancer Society, ME Division, Inc., 52 Federal Street, Brunswick, ME 04011. For children and adolescents 7 and up who have or have had cancer and their families. Free.

CAMP SUNSHINE
Contact: Point Sebago
Outdoor Resort, RR #1, Box
712, Casco, ME 04015. 207-
655-3821. Family program,
four one-week overnight
camps. Free.

MASSACHUSETTS
CAMP CAROL
Contact: Dr. & Mrs. Bill
Egan, 87 Redlands Road,
West Roxbury, MA 02132.
617-327-1913. Three one-
week summer sessions at
Lake Winnepisaukee for
children 8–15 with cancer.
Free.

MICHIGAN
CAMP QUALITY—
MICHIGAN
Jeanne Rossman,
Administrative Director, 308
East Hibbard Road, Owosso,
MI 48867. 517-723-2553.
Sponsor: Reorganized
Church of Jesus Christ of
Latter Day Saints. For
children with cancer. Free.

SPECIAL DAYS CAMP
Contact: George L. Royer,
MD, Executive Medical
Director, or Carole J. Royer,
Camp Director, P.O. Box
174, Portage, MI 49081.
616-344-4911. Overnight
one- and two-week summer
sessions for children with

cancer on or off therapy and
cured. Special Days Partners
program for siblings 8–18.
Winter program for both.
$20.00-$125.00; financial
assistance.

MINNESOTA
CAMP COURAGE
Contact: Courage Center,
Camping Department, 3915
Golden Valley Road, Golden
Valley, MN 55422.
612-588-0811. Six-day session
for children 6–13; six-day
session for teens.

CAMP K.A.C.E. (KIDS
AGAINST CANCER
EVERYWHERE) Contact:
Greg Diehl/Robert Larson,
Lake Agassiz Camp Fire
Council, Inc., 725 Center
Avenue, Moorhead, MN
56560. 218-236-1090.
Overnight camp for children
with cancer and siblings
7–20. $25.00 per family;
financial assistance.

MISSISSIPPI
CAMP RAINBOW
Contact: Pam Dotson,
American Cancer Society,
MS Division, Inc., 1380
Livingston Lane, Jackson,
MS 39213-8013.
601-362-8874. For children
6–19 who have or have had
cancer. Three-day overnight
camp weekend. Free.

MISSOURI
CAMP QUALITY
NORTHWEST MISSOURI
Contact: Kay Jensen,
Director, Barnard, MO
64423, 816-652-3218, or
Edwin or Lavina Jones,
Co-directors, 1301
Savannah, Mound City, MO
64470, 816-442-5668.
Sponsor: Reorganized
Church of Jesus Christ of
Latter Day Saints. One-week
session for children with
cancer, pre-school to 21, in
special situations, siblings.

CAMP QUALITY OZARK
MISSOURI
Contact: Cheryl Henning,
Director, Rt. 2, Box 497,
Joplin, MO 64304, or Janet
Ramsey, Co-director, Rt. 7,
Box 300-8, Springfield, MO
65802. 417-865-4669.
Sponsor: Reorganized
Church of Jesus Christ of
Latter Day Saints. For
children with cancer. Free.

CAMP SHAWNEE
Contact: Kansas City,
Missouri, Council of Camp
Fire, 8733 Sni-a-Bar Road,
Kansas City, MO 64129.
816-737-3256. Overnight
camp for children 6–17 with
cancer. Free.

CAMP SUNRISE
Contact: American Cancer
Society, MO Division, Inc.,
3322 American Avenue, P.O.
Box 1066, Jefferson City,
MO 65101. Weekend for
families with a child 8 or
younger who has cancer.

KIWANIS CAMP WYMAN
Contact: Mary Dwyer,
Director, 600 Kiwanis Drive,
Eureka, MO 63025. 314-938-
5245. Eleven-day summer
program for children 8–16;
mainstreams children with
cancer into the regular
program. Financial
assistance.

NEBRASKA
CAMP CO HO LO
(COURAGE, HOPE &
LOVE)
Contact: Aniza Lerum, RN,
Oncology/Hematology,
Children's Hospital,
402-390-5400, or Robyn
Freeman, Camp Fire
Council, Inc., 1805 Harney
Street, Omaha, NE 68102,
402-345-2491. For children
with cancer 6–17. $10.00.

NEW JERSEY
CAMP HAPPY TIMES
Contact: Emy Hyans, Valerie
Fund Children's Center,
Overlook Hospital, Summit,
NJ 07901. 201-522-2353.

One-week camp for New Jersey children 6–16 who are or have been treated for cancer. *Camp Happy Times Teen Experience* for 16–19-year-olds with cancer. Free. Transportation available.

HAPPINESS IS CAMPING
Contact: Murray Struver, 2169 Grand Concourse, Bronx, NY 10453. 212-295-3100. Mailing address: Happiness Is Camping, 62 Sunset Lake Road, Blairstown, NJ 07825. Multi-length sessions for children with cancer. Free.

NEW YORK
CAMP GOOD DAYS & SPECIAL TIMES, INC.
Contact: Camp Good Days & Special Times, Inc., 100 White Spruce Boulevard, Rochester, NY 14623. 716-427-2650. Several programs: (1) Camp Good Days: residential camp for children 7–18 with cancer; (2) Junior Good Days: four-day program for children 4–7, in Buffalo, Rochester, and Syracuse; (3) Brothers & Sisters Together (Camp B.E.S.T.): a year-round support program for siblings who have or have had a brother or sister with cancer, culminating in a summer residential camping experience; (4) Moms & Pops: residential camp for parents who have or have had a child with cancer; (5) Childhood U.S.A. (Understanding, Support, and Assistance): a year-round support program for children who have or have had a parent with cancer, culminating in a summer residential camping experience.

CAMP OPEN ARMS
Contact: Cancer Action, 1441 East Avenue, Rochester, NY 14610. 716-473-8230. Two-week day camp for children 3–15 with cancer and blood diseases and their siblings. Free.

CAMP SIMCHA
Contact: Devorah Lipson, Program Director, Camp Simcha, c/o Chai Lifeline, 5323 12th Avenue, Brooklyn, NY 11219. 718-436-7373. One-week kosher camp for Jewish children 7–20 who have cancer or other life-threatening illnesses. Free.

MID-HUDSON VALLEY
CAMP
Contact: Mid-Hudson Valley
Camp, Esopus, NY 12429,
914-384-6620, or Ms. Naomi
Schrenzel, CSW,
212-305-7786. One-week
camp for children with
cancer. Free.

NORTH CAROLINA
CAMP CARE
Contact: Mrs. Lynn Dobson,
Camp Director, P.O. Box
35072, Charlotte, NC 28235.
704-399-3465. Overnight
camping trip for children 6–
16 who are in treatment for
cancer, in relapse, remission,
or cancer free. Counselors
are all former cancer
patients. Free.

NORTH CAROLINA
CAMP CAREFREE
Contact: Anne Jones, Rt. 2,
Box 322A, Stokesdale, NC
27357. 919-427-0966. For
children 7–17 with cancer
and chronic illnesses.
Different sessions, one also
for siblings. Free, first to
children from North Carolina
and out-of-state children
treated in North Carolina.

CAMP RAINBOW
Contact: Jacque Price, Child/
Family Specialist, East
Carolina University School of
Medicine, Pediatric
Hematology & Oncology,
PCMH 288 West,
Greenville, NC 27834-4354.
919-515-4676. One-week
program supported by Pitt
County United Way and
Medical Foundation of East
Carolina University. For
children 6–18 with cancer
and their siblings. Children
who have lost a sibling to
cancer are also encouraged
to attend. Free to children
from eastern North Carolina.

OHIO
CAMP FRIENDSHIP
Contact: American Cancer
Society, OH Division, Inc.,
5555 Frantz Road, Dublin,
OH 43017. 614-889-9565.
Two four- and one-half day
sessions, at YMCA Camp
Kern in southern Ohio, and
at Hiram House Camp in
northern Ohio. Ages 7–15.
Free.

KIDS 'N KAMP
Contact: Beverly S. Circone,
Executive Director, 1035
West Third Avenue,
Columbus, OH 43212.
614-299-0316. Fall camp

weekend, spring family picnic, October pumpkin hunt & hay ride, holiday parties. For children with cancer or other blood diseases and their families. Free.

OKLAHOMA
CAMP FUN IN THE SUN & FUN IN THE FALL
Contact: Pat Schenoor, SW, Oklahoma Children's Memorial Hospital, 940 Northeast 13th, Oklahoma City, OK 73104. 405-271-4412. For children in therapy only. Friday to Sunday program. Free.

CAMP WALUHILI
Contact: Sherry Rose, Director of Camping Services, Camp Fire, Inc., 5305 East 41st, Tulsa, OK 74135. 918-663-3443. Special half-week session for children 6–17 with cancer and one of their siblings 7–17. Free.

OREGON
CAMP UKANDU
Contact: Ken Raddle, American Cancer Society, OR Division, Inc., 0330 Southwest Curry Street, Portland, OR 97201. 503-295-6422. Located in Yamhill, Oregon. For children with cancer 9–18 and their siblings.

PENNSYLVANIA
CAMP CAN-DO
Contact: American Cancer Society, PA Division, Rt. 422 & Sipe Avenue, Hershey, PA 17033. 717-533-6144. For children 8–18 who are in or have had treatment for cancer.

CAMP DOST
Contact: Paul Kettlewell, PhD, Geisinger Medical Center, Danville, PA 17822. 717-271-8255. One-week summer program for cancer children 5–18.

RONALD McDONALD CAMP
Contact: Patricia Boyle, Camp Administrator, Ronald McDonald House, 3925 Chestnut Street, Philadelphia, PA 19104. 215-387-8406 or 215-596-9608 (messages). For kids with cancer who have had treatment or are undergoing treatment at the Children's Hospital of Philadelphia. Free.

RHODE ISLAND
CAMP HOPE
Contact: American Cancer Society, RI Division, 400 Main Street, Pawtucket, RI

02860. 800-662-5000. One-week overnight camp for children with cancer living in or treated in Rhode Island. Free.

SOUTH CAROLINA
CAMP KEMO
Contact: Beth Coleman, Camp Director, Children's Hospital, Richland Memorial Center for Cancer and Blood Disorders, 5 Richland Medical Park, Columbia, SC 29203. 803-765-6484. One-week overnight camp for children and adolescents 5–18 with cancer and one sibling 7–16 from South Carolina. Teens accepted as counselors. Free.

CAMP HAPPY DAYS
Contact: Debby Stephenson, P.O. Box 2154, Summerville, SC 29484. 803-873-8072. Free. Ages 5–18.

TENNESSEE
CAMP EAGLE NEST
Contact: Child Life Director, East Tennessee Children's Hospital, P.O. Box 15010, Knoxville, TN 37901. 615-544-3448. One-week overnight camp.

CAMP HORIZON
Contact: Leila Rust, Director of Medical Affairs, American Cancer Society, TN Division, Inc., 1315 8th Avenue South, Nashville, TN 37203. 615-383-1710. One-week overnight camp.

TEXAS
CAMP RAINBOW CONNECTION
Contact: Ruth Anne Herring, RN, UTMB, Rt. C-61, Galveston, TX 77550. 409-761-2341. For children 6–17 who are or have been treated at the University of Texas Medical Branch. $5.00 registration fee.

CANDLELIGHTERS CAMP COURAGEOUS
Contact: Susan Lee/Robyn Tomas, University Towers, Suite 206A, 1900 North Oregon Street, El Paso, TX 79902. 915-544-2222. For children 6–19 with cancer. Free on a first-come, first-served basis.

CAMP DISCOVERY
Contact: Karen Torges, American Cancer Society, Medical Affairs, 8214 Wurzbach Road, San Antonio, TX 78229. 512-696-4211. Children 6–18. Free.

CAMP ESPERANZA
Contact: Peggy Sartain, MD, Children's Medical Center, Department of Pediatrics, 5323 Harry Hines, Dallas, TX 75235. 214-920-2382. Children 6–15 treated at the center. Free.

CAMP PERIWINKLE
Contact: Judy H. Packler, CSW, Research Hematology Department, Texas Children's Hospital, 6621 Fannin, Houston, TX 77030. 713-791-4122. Children 7–16 treated at Texas Children's Hospital. One sibling invited on a space-available basis. Free.

CAMP SANGUINITY
Contact: Penny Bennett, RN, Cook-Fort Worth Children's Medical Center, 1212 West Lancaster, Fort Worth, TX 76102. 817-336-5521. For children 6–16 with cancer or blood disorders treated at Cook and their siblings. One week resident camp. Free.

CAMP STAR TRAILS
Contact: Janet Johnson, RN, Pediatrics, University of Texas, M.D. Anderson Hospital, 1515 Holcombe, Houston TX 77030. 713-792-2465. Children and their siblings 5–14 from M.D. Anderson and state of Texas. One-week overnight camp. $60.00; camperships.

UTAH
CAMP HOBE
Contact: American Cancer Society, UT Division, Inc., 610 East South Temple, Salt Lake City, UT 84102. 801-322-0431. For children with cancer and their siblings.

VERMONT
CAMP TA-KUM-TA
Contact: Ted Kessler, American Cancer Society, VT Division, Inc., Camp Ta-Kum-Ta, P.O. Box 576, Waterbury, VT 05676, 802-479-2253. For children 7-17 with cancer. Free.

VIRGINIA
CAMP FANTASTIC
Contact: David A. Smith, Executive Director, Special Love, Inc., P.O. Box 3243, Winchester, VA 22601. 703-662-2270. One-week overnight camp for children 7–17 with cancer from

National Cancer Institute, District of Columbia Children's Hospital, Georgetown, Johns Hopkins, University of Virginia, MCV, Walter Reed, Kings Daughters.

CAMP FIVE SEASONS
Contact: Patricia Holden, Executive Director, 3704 Farnsworth Drive, Chesapeake, VA 23321. 804-484-0984 or 804-547-5145. Overnight camp for healthy and medically challenged children and their siblings 7–14. $150.00; scholarships. Limit of 49 children per session.

CAMP HOLIDAY TRAILS
Contact: Camp Holiday Trails, P.O. Box 5806, Charlottesville, VA. 22906-0806. 804-977-3781. Therapeutic residential summer camp for children 7–17 with medical and physical health needs including cancer. Two two-week sessions ($375 each) and one three-week session ($550). Also one- to three-day therapeutic programs in the fall, winter, and spring, i.e.

disabled skiing instruction, ages 7 to adult. Financial assistance.

WASHINGTON
CAMP GOODTIMES WEST/CAMP GOODTIMES EAST
Contact: Ms. Pamela M. Smith, Program Director, American Cancer Society, WA Division, Inc., 2120 1st Avenue North, Seattle, WA 98109. 206-283-1152. American Cancer Society, Spokane Unit. 509-326-5802. Two summer camps: Camp Goodtimes West on Vashon Island, and Camp Goodtimes East near Spokane. For children with cancer and their siblings from Washington. Free.

CANADA
CAMP OOCHIGEAS
Contact: Louise Heinrich, Camp Secretary, Camp Oochigeas, 366 Glencairn Avenue, Toronto, Ontario, Canada M5N 1V1. 416-482-4122. Sponsored by Toronto Ronald McDonald House. For children 7 and up who have or have had cancer. Two-week and one-week sessions. Limited financial assistance.

CAMP QUALITY ONTARIO
Contact: Eunic Taylor,
Director, 58 Bay Hill Drive,
Concord, Ontario L4K 1G9,
Canada, 416-738-9994, or
Becky Shantz, Assistant
Director, Box 165, Aur,
Ontario N0B 1E0, Canada.
Sponsor: Reorganized
Church of Jesus Christ of
Latter Day Saints. For
children with cancer. Free.

AUSTRALIA
CAMP QUALITY
Contact: Vera Entwistle,
President, Camp Quality, 5
Taylor Street, West Pennant
Hills 2120, NSW, Australia.
02-872-5454. Sponsor:
Reorganized Church of Jesus
Christ of Latter Day Saints.
For children with cancer.
Free.

Is there any organization that can help me get my medical records?

If you want to see or get a copy of your medical records, ask the hospital, doctor, or other member of the medical team. If they will not give the records to you, try asking another doctor to get them for you. The first doctor (or the hospital) usually has to give your records to another doctor who asks for them.

About half of the states have laws giving you the right to see your medical records. The laws vary greatly, with some giving you access to both doctor and hospital records and others covering only hospital records. (Most also have laws protecting confidentiality and access to mental health records). You can get information about the laws in your state by writing to the American Medical Record Association, Office of Legislative Affairs, 875 North Michigan Avenue, Chicago, IL 60611, or by calling 312-787-2672.

If your records are at a federal facility, a Veterans Administration Hospital, Public Health Service facility, or a military hospital under the Department of Defense, they are covered by the federal Freedom of Information Act and Privacy Act. This should make it easier for you to see the records, since requests under either act are to be answered or acknowledged within ten working days.

Are there any consumer organizations that deal with insurance issues?

Yes. The National Insurance Consumer Organization is a nonprofit public interest advocacy and educational organization which promotes the interests of insurance buyers and helps consumers buy insurance wisely. You can write 121 North Payne Street, Alexandria, VA 22314, or call 703-549-8050.

The People's Medical Society (14 East Minor Street, Emmaus, PA 18049), which acts as a consumer advocate in the health-care field, is also involved in helping consumers evaluate and select health insurance.

Your local social security office distributes single copies of a Guide to Health Insurance for People with Medicare, which explains what Medicare does not pay for and what to look for in private health insurance.

The American Council of Life Insurance, an industry association, has a library which includes its publications along with those of the Health Insurance Association of America and other health-related organizations. A bibliography of materials may be obtained free of charge by writing 1850 K Street, NW, Washington, DC, or by calling 800-423-8000.

What advocacy groups deal with women's health problems?

The National Women's Health Network is a national consumer group devoted to women and their health needs. They are concerned with rights of women in health care and in helping understand cancer. The organization headquarters is at 224 7th Street, SE, Washington, DC 20003; telephone: 202-347-1140.

The Boston Women's Health Book Collective, Inc., in West Summerville, ME (617-625-0271), is a health information center involved in numerous women's health education and advocacy projects.

The Women's Occupational Health Resource Center is a non-profit organization dedicated to workplace health and safety. The group is located at Columbia University, School of Public Health and Comprehensive Cancer Center, 21 Audubon Avenue, 3rd Floor, New York, NY 10032; telephone: 718-230-8822.

The Women's Breast Advisory Center, 11426 Rockville Pike, Rockville, MD 20850, founded by Rose Kushner, provides information on all aspects of breast disease, especially cancer.

Do any of the advocacy groups for older citizens deal with cancer issues?

Most of them do. There are several you can contact if you have specific consumer problems you need to discuss. Among them:

- American Association of Retired Persons, Health Advocacy Services, 1909 K Street, NW, Washington, DC 20049. The Association encourages the effective use of the health-care system by older Americans and offers detailed information on Medicare, guidelines for shopping for supplemental insurance, information on the advantages and disadvantages of Health Maintenance Organizations, and their relationship with Medicare.
- Legal Counsel for the Elderly, P.O. Box 19269K, Washington, DC 20036, informs individuals about legal rights around the issues of Medicare and other health problems.
- Inspector General's Hotline of the Department of Health and Human Services (1-800-368-5779) handles complaints and assists consumers who have been overbilled or billed for services not rendered by Medicare and Medicaid.
- The Gray Panthers National Office (31 South Juniper Street, Philadelphia, PA 19107; telephone: 215-545-6555), National Council on the Aging (600 Maryland Avenue, SW, West Wing 100, Washington, DC 20024), and the National Caucus and Center on Black Aged (1424 K Street, NW, Washington, DC 20005; telephone: 202-637-8400) may also be helpful.

Are there consumer groups dealing with cancer and the environment or the workplace?

There are several groups working in those areas, including:
- The Environmental Law Institute (1616 P Street, NW, 2nd Floor, Washington, DC 20036; telephone: 202-328-5150)—a non-profit, national research center dedicated to the design of effective environmental policies and the improvement of institutional abilities to implement existing law and policy, also seeks to develop innovative and improved strategies for controlling hazardous substances.
- Sierra Club (730 Polk Street, San Francisco, CA 94109; telephone: 415-776-2211)—a nationwide environmental organization with over 350,000 members, focuses on effecting changes in federal and state laws in the area of reducing exposure to carcinogens.
- Southwest Research and Information Center (P.O. Box 4524, Albuquerque, NM 87106; telephone: 505-262-1862) —a non-profit organization providing information on environmental and social issues throughout the country.
- The American Labor Education Center (1835 Kilbourne Place, NW, Washington, DC 20010; telephone: 202-387-6780)—an independent, non-profit educational institution which provides printed and audiovisual materials on specific hazards, including carcinogens in the wood-products industry.

What is the American Council on Science and Health?

This is a scientific, consumer-education organization directed by a panel of 80 scientists, physicians, and policy advisors. The American Council on Science and Health provides accurate, balanced information on health-related topics, such as asbestos and estrogen. (1995 Broadway, 18th Floor, New York, NY 10023; telephone: 212-362-7044.)

What does the Office on Smoking and Health do?

It is an office of the federal government, serving as a central source of scientific and technical information about smoking. It develops the annual *Surgeon General's Report on Smoking* and provides consumer-oriented information. Its data bank has thousands of articles on smoking. (Office on Smoking and Health, Park Building, 5600 Fishers Lane, Rockville, MD 20857.)

Are there groups taking advocacy stands in the area of food and nutrition?

Several groups are working on these issues, including:
- The Center for Science in the Public Interest (1501 16th Street, NW, Washington, DC 20036)—works to strengthen laws that regulate the use of food additives and ingredients, require food additives and other chemicals to be tested for their effects on human behavior and mental health, halt deceptive advertising, prevent alcohol abuse and alcoholism, and investigate the marketing practices of the alcoholic beverage industry. This private non-profit organization also publishes a variety of educational materials for the general public on the topics of nutrition, health, and science.
- The Community Nutrition Institute (2001 South Street, NW, Suite 530, Washington, DC 20009; telephone: 202-462-4700)—a non-profit, citizen organization specializing in food and nutrition issues at the community and legislative level, also offers a publications list of printed materials.

In addition, there are several groups sponsored by the food industry, including:
- The United Fresh Fruit and Vegetable Association (727 North Washington, Alexandria, VA 22314; telephone:

703-836-4310)—promotes the use of fresh fruits and vegetables in a well-balanced diet.

• National Dairy Council (6300 North River Road, Rose-
mont, IL 60618; telephone: 312-696-1020)—an educational and scientific organization funded by the dairy
industry, encouraging food selection patterns that include
dairy foods and other major food categories in accordance
with scientific recommendations.

Where can I get articles on cancer subjects?

Articles which appear in the most popular non-technical
magazines and journals are listed in the *Readers' Guide to
Periodical Literature* or in the *Public Affairs Information
Service*. These are usually available in most public libraries.
Look in the index under the subject in which you are inter-
ested—or if you know it, under the author's name.

Where can I find articles which are in health–science jour-
nals?

The *Index Medicus*, which is found in medical libraries, most
university and college libraries, and some public libraries,
lists articles appearing in over 2,600 science journals. The
National Library of Medicine has created a family of medical
databases called MEDLARS, which include the following:

MEDLINE, with more than four million citations and
abstracts of approximately 3,200 medical journals published
in the United States and throughout the world.

PDQ, or Physician Date Query, which has been discussed
earlier.

CANCERLIT, with approximately 550,000 citations and
abstracts of articles published since 1978 on all aspects of
cancer.

Index

In the process of reading and using this book, questions which are not included in it may come to your mind. The authors would be most pleased if you would share your thoughts with them.

Kindly send any comments to:

Eve Potts, Marion Morra
c/o Avon Books
105 Madison Avenue
New York, NY 10016

MARION MORRA is the Assistant Director of the Yale Comprehensive Cancer Center at the Yale University School of Medicine in New Haven, Connecticut. She is also Associate Clinical Professor at the Yale School of Nursing, teaching graduate-level classes in communications and health marketing. Marion is widely published, having written articles and authored books for both the health profession and the public, with emphasis on health and especially in the field of cancer. She serves on several major national committees for the National Cancer Institute and the American Cancer Society.

EVE POTTS has been a medical writer for more than 30 years. Her expertise is in making difficult medical information easy to understand. She has been Director of Advertising and Medical Education for Spencer, Incorporated, served as a medical writer and consultant to the Department of Health and Human Services, written medical monographs for drug companies, and served as a writer and consultant for a wide variety of medical institutions.

The two authors, who are sisters, have collaborated on two other books: *CHOICES: Realistic Alternatives in Cancer Treatment* (Avon Books, 1980, revised ed. 1987) and *Understanding Your Immune System* (Avon Books, 1986). They live and work in Connecticut.

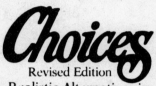